P9-APW-598

DATE DUE

FEB 20 '85			
APR 23 '86			
DEC 27 1989			
JAN 8 1992			
AP 10 '96			

170 IDEAL   PRINTED IN U.S.A.

QUEST BOOKS
are published by
The Theosophical Society in America,
a branch of a world organization
dedicated to the promotion of brotherhood and
the encouragement of the study of religion,
philosophy, and science, to the end that man may
better understand himself and his place in
the universe. The Society stands for complete
freedom of individual search and belief.
In the Theosophical Classics Series
well-known occult works are made
available in popular editions.

Cover design by Kathy Miners

HEALTH:
A HOLISTIC APPROACH

How to maintain a state of health
in body, mind, and spirit.

**DENNIS CHERNIN, M.D. and
GREGORY MANTEUFFEL, M.D.**

WITHDRAWN
by Unity Library

UNITY SCHOOL LIBRARY
UNITY VILLAGE, MISSOURI 64065

*This publication made possible with
the assistance of the Kern Foundation*

The Theosophical Publishing House
Wheaton, Ill. U.S.A.
Madras, India/London, England

© Copyright by Dennis Chernin and Gregory Manteuffel
A Quest original. First edition 1984.
All rights reserved.
No part of this book may be reproduced in any manner
without written permission except for quotations embodied
in critical articles or reviews.

For additional information write to:
The Theosophical Publishing House
306 West Geneva Road
Wheaton, Illinois 60189

Published by The Theosophical Publishing House,
a department of The Theosophical Society in America.

Library of Congress Cataloging in Publication Data

Chernin, Dennis, 1949-
    Health: a holistic approach.

    11-84

    "A Quest book"
    Bibliography: p.
    Includes index.
    1. Holistic medicine.   2. Health.   3. Mind and body.
4. Yoga.   I. Manteuffel, Gregory, 1948-   II. Title
R723.C44   1984   613   84-402070
ISBN 0-8356-0590-6 (pbk.)

Printed in the United States of America

Contents

Acknowledgments

We would like to extend our appreciation to Barbara Bova for helping to organize and edit this book. Special thanks goes to Chris Schmidt for his precise illustrations and to Matthew Monsein, M.D., and Ed Funk, M.D., for their medical consultations. Other important contributions came from Linda Johnsen for typing, Patricia Williams-Gross for final typing, and Kathy Marien for additional editing.

A personal thanks goes to Dennis Chernin's wife Jan and their sons, Abraham, Ethan, and and the late Nathaniel, whose understanding, patience, and love inspired his writing.

I

Introduction to Holistic Medicine

1

The Holistic Perspective

Sensitivity to the order, beauty and balance of nature evokes a sense of oneness that can only be felt and not measured. Because we are also manifestations of the natural world, we are subject to the same forces that influence all patterns and aspects of the universe. It makes sense to take these forces into account in medicine, the science of health, since the rules that govern health are also part of this natural order.

As physicians, we have been given the opportunity to explore the meaning of health and disease. Our traditional medical training, with all the sophistication that modern technology provides, has helped us to understand anatomy, physiology, biochemistry, and pathology. However, it was necessary to expand that knowledge in order to gain a greater understanding of the seemingly subtle influences that underlie the body's physiochemistry and orchestrate integration of the human being. It was the desire to integrate our scientific training with that which can only be experienced intuitively and instinctively that led us to explore philosophical systems which have their roots in the order of nature. It was our feeling that modern medicine has done well in treating many illnesses and containing infectious

3

diseases but has not gone far enough in defining and teaching the principles of health and creating an atmosphere of wholeness. We wished to explore systems of health care, both modern and ancient, which facilitated an understanding that body, mind, and spirit are interdependent.

We began to realize that holism does not necessarily imply alternative modes of treatment, for these methods can often be superficial, nonverifiable, or unidimensional. Nor did it imply that traditional physicians could not be holistic. What seemed to be most important was for the practitioner of holism to create an atmosphere where mind and body are seen to be interconnected and the psychological and spiritual dimensions of physical illnesses are consistently acknowledged.

Initially, the study of ancient and other holistic systems seemed overwhelming and confusing and exposed such a multitude of available techniques that underlying perspectives were not immediately apparent. However, as our research progressed, commonalities surfaced, revealing unifying principles behind the fundamental teachings of the different medical and philosophical systems. These principles which are re-addressed throughout this book, include:

(1) A fundamental acceptance of man's *integrated nature* as a spiritual mental, emotional, and physical being.[1] Health and disease can best be assessed with complete knowledge as to the degree of restriction on each of these levels of human functioning. This view contrasts with the belief system of modern scientific medicine which is largely Descartian in its assumption that there is a dualistic relationship between the separate and distinct entities of mind and body. Accordingly, diseases which are manifest mostly in the physical level are diagnosed and treated with little or no consideration as to mental and emotional health.

---

[1]The word *man* is used in this book in its generic sense meaning humanity, including women. The pronouns *he*, *him*, *his* are used for convenience and are also meant to include the female of the species.

(2) A *vitalistic view* of medicine which implies that the processes of life cannot be explained by the laws of physics and chemistry alone, but that life is in some part endowed with the power of enduring or continuing. Since this power of enduring, or vitality, cannot be readily measured by the physical sciences, it is largely disregarded in modern scientific medicine. In holistic medicine systems, however, it is understood that this vitality forms the very foundation for sound mental, emotional, and physical well-being and strengthening of the vitality results in heightened resistance to disease. This vitality keeps the human being alive and underlies the body's defense mechanisms. It operates outside of everyday waking consciousness and is thus called the body's innate intelligence.

(3) A *philosophic perspective* to medicine to help free thinking from the rigid constraints imposed by physical scientific methodology, thus allowing mankind to search broadly in pursuit of wisdom and facilitate the integration of spirituality and medicine.

(4) An orientation toward *personal growth* which results from the individual taking responsibility for maintaining health and overcoming susceptibility to disease. Holistic systems guide a person to expand his awareness concerning himself and his environment through the examination of attitudes, feelings, and habits which undermine vitality and predispose him to disease. The knowledge that is gained in this process helps one feel more powerful and less victimized by illness and is fundamental to understanding the basic universal phenomena of cause and effect.

(5) A realization of the *balance and unity* that exists between man and nature. Man is a part of nature and is subject to its laws. If he chooses to follow these laws, he may experience relative harmony as he explores the mysteries of life. On the other hand, if natural laws are rejected, man can feel victimized by the consequences of such a choice and life may seem hostile and cruel.

(6) A sense of *community* which is especially fostered by ancient holistic systems by addressing the issue of spiritual

growth, with emphasis on such concepts as improving the quality of existence, experiencing the unity of all things, and practicing true compassion toward others. On a more mundane level this includes living in harmony with the earth and preserving the quality of the environment for the generations to come.

There are ways and means to seek truth, growth, balance, contentment, and health common to all the systems, but these are presented differently. These varying perspectives served to increase our clarity of observation and enrich our understanding. We finally concluded that all of the holistic systems are complementary and synergistic. The various systems can be likened to the spokes which emanate from the central hub of a wheel. The hub is symbolic of the natural order of which the human being is a manifestation. Each spoke represents a unique interpretation of the dynamics of this order. That the spokes resemble one another is understandable, as their origin is the same.

As a result of this research, we have written this book, emphasizing the common principles which underlie all truly holistic and natural systems of therapy. We have found that being involved in any one facet of the holistic health movement, whether it be nutrition, acupuncture, hatha yoga, body work, or meditation, leads to an understanding that can be easily integrated with other holistic practices.

The roots of holistic medicine are ancient. Systems of healing that integrate the areas of body, mind, and spirit developed over thousands of years in the East. Modern holistic therapies have adopted many of their principles from the Indian systems of yoga and Ayurveda and from Chinese medicine. By integrating ancient ideas of the East with modern Western biochemical and technological knowledge, the foundation for holistic medicine treatment has been built. It is this synthesis of the East with the West which can help us in the modern world to overcome health problems and to utilize our fullest potentials to live creatively as fully integrated individuals.

In this book we have attempted to discuss only those principles, theories, and techniques that we use in our own general medical practice. We have tried to maintain our integrity by not presenting information that is impractical or superficial. The systems described are all either time-tested, such as the more ancient systems of Chinese medicine, Ayurveda, and yoga philosophy, or are scientifically verified, including the modern therapies of nutrition, psychotherapy, homeopathy, and stress management. We have emphasized yoga philosophy as our primary holistic preventive model and have used it as the integrating system. This is not because we believe that it is the epitome of holistic paradigms but because it offers a readily available system, therapeutically and philosophically. It offers a cogent, concise, and sophisticated theoretical framework through which other therapies can be integrated and systematized. Also, on a more pragmatic level, we ourselves practice the techniques and disciplines of yoga, both in the medical profession and in our own daily individual lives, and therefore we are more familiar with its intricacies.

Our choice of yoga as the emphasis in this book, of course, does not preclude the validity of other holistic models. Other systems such as Chinese medicine or Ayurveda are equally complete, but we have not studied these in as much detail as yoga. For this reason, these two sections are less developed in our book. We have chosen to present Ayurveda and Chinese medicine generally as theoretical models and less as therapeutic systems. We do not often use the herbs found in these great schools of medicine nor do we use pulse diagnosis or acupuncture extensively. Yet, we do use their principles in understanding the individual patient. We find that the theoretical perspective found in Chinese and Ayurvedic medicine complement all the other systems and help us appreciate, in a more complete manner, disease and health.

We realize that there are some sections in this book that may appear general and oversimplified, such as nutrition, homeopathy, and psychotherapy. Each of these subjects can fill many textbooks with detail and specificity. Our purpose is simply to indicate that we use these approaches in our practice and also, more important, to exemplify how they, like the more ancient systems, help us see with clarity the whole patient. For example, we have avoided duplication of the many popular diets and diverse approaches to nutrition but have attempted to show that many holistic systems operate through a nutritional perspective.

Because all the information presented here is used in our practice, we have taken the liberty not to document scientifically all the statements made. We have footnoted some of the modern nutritional areas that have been proven with rigorous testing. However, it is a much harder task to demonstrate with precision the source of more generalized ideas because the principles and techniques have been stated and restated in so many places and times. Empirical proof that is substantiated through years of use by millions of people is a form of validation. The extensive bibliography can provide much useful information and guidance towards the many sources of this great pool of knowledge.

There are two major audiences to whom we address this book. The first is physicians and health practitioners who are interested in understanding principles of holism in medicine. While many books have been written outlining various models, we feel we offer a concise model that can be used not only to understand holistic medicine theoretically but also to be used therapeutically. It is a truly integrative approach illustrating how all the modalities we employ in our practice can be used in a unified manner. The other group we have attempted to reach is the lay public. This book can serve the purpose of helping to add clarity to confusion in the mushrooming field of holistic medicine. It offers a practical framework not only to help a person understand the nature of health from a body-mind-spirit perspective but also to understand and treat oneself during illness. For the latter purpose, we have included an appendix to teach people some of the techniques of yoga and some basic relaxation techniques.

The first part of this book is an introduction to the concept of holistic medicine. The second part examines the roots of holistic medicine with an overview of three ancient medical systems: Chinese, Ayurvedic, and yogic. The third part of the book is an analysis of modern holistic models. The last part is an overview using the system of yoga philosophy as a practical framework around which a holistic approach can be organized. Five diseases are then discussed in terms of both theory and treatment. In these cases all the ancient and modern holistic systems previously discussed are integrated.

2

Theory and Principles
of Holistic Medicine

According to the concept of *holistic medicine*, health and wholeness imply the integration of the physical, mental, and spiritual levels of being. From this perspective, man is more than a machine that can be serviced like the family automobile. He is a person with spiritual and social aspects whose well-being is as much a reflection of the health of his psyche as it is a reflection of his physical health. Man is meant to function as a totally integrated being, and any medical system of analysis or diagnosis that effectively treats him must also be complete. As we search for ways to achieve health and prevent illness, holistic or preventive medical systems are slowly beginning to flourish.

Before delving into the various therapies utilized in holistic medicine, it is first necessary to redefine the concept of health. From a holistic perspective, *health* is not merely the absence of disease. Being healthy implies that an individual is capable of positively adapting to changes in inner and outer environments. Health is not a static phenomenon but a dynamic process reflecting a positive physical and mental adjustment to varying stressful circumstances. These stresses can assume many different forms: emotional upheaval, climatic events, microbial infestation, or enervating habits of one's life style. Being healthy does not mean a person never feels mental or physical pain, but that he is able to put them in perspective, can learn from the experience and continue to grow. He is free to experience the full gamut of emotions but does not become enslaved by them.

In accordance with this definition of health, *symptoms* represent the organism's attempt to re-establish homeostasis and well-being and are thus informative and protective. Healthy people view their symptomatology positively, as a tool and as feedback that something is amiss internally. Many physical symptoms can be understood to be the body's attempt to eliminate waste or toxins, as exemplified by boils, eczema, or mucous membrane discharges. Mental and emotional symptoms can be viewed as the psyche's attempt to bring emotional repressions to the surface. A person practicing holistic medicine tries to live simply, with awareness, and is open to exploring the underlying causes of his illness.

Cause of Disease

When a person achieves a relative balance of body, mind, and spirit, he is living holistically and harmoniously. Maintaining harmony also means that he is constantly in the process of preventing illness. This harmony is disturbed when a person's inner state is characterized by overemotionalism, aimlessness, negative thought patterns, or lack of spiritual direction. When these conditions are reinforced by disturbing habits, such as poor nutrition, lack of exercise, or stimulant abuse, the result is a weakened organism, which is susceptible to disease. Thus, from this viewpoint, the microbial world is merely the exciting cause of disease that preys on a devitalized spirit, mind, body, and immune system, and the actual cause of disease is considered to originate within man's mental and emotional spheres. *Disease* can thus be defined as the inability to adapt properly to the ever-changing stresses and vicissitudes of life, so that dissipating and negative habits predominate. The ailing person may resent being ill, would like to simply eliminate the symptoms without ever understanding the underlying causes, and in general retains a morbid fear of sickness.

It is obvious that the system of holistic medicine involves a reorientation of the way in which Western medicine is accustomed to viewing health and disease and the cause and prevention of disease. The philosophy of Western man is materialistic; his reality is largely governed by physical laws. Western medicine perceives the cause of disease similarly. It limits itself to exploring only those factors which can be understood and categorized by physical laws. Subjective or intuitive knowledge cannot be readily measured and, except for the study of a few diseases considered to be psychosomatic, is largely disregarded. To a large extent, then, Western man has cut himself off from inner knowledge or guidance which tells him that he is part of a greater whole. Without this knowledge, man feels alienated from his environment, and rather than flowing with nature, he tries to control it. A "me against them" intellect is the result of this loss of attunement with nature. He thus has the tendency to blame external phenomena such as the weather, bacteria, or stress for his ills. As a result, prevention of disease has generally been oriented around control and eradication of these presumed causal factors.

Besides infectious agents (bacteria and viruses), Western medicine acknowledges several other categories of disease causation. These include: (1) genetics or inherited problems; (2) deficiency disorders, such as nutritional or endocrine imbalances; (3) neoplastic or tumor growths; (4) inflammatory processes characterized by swelling and heat; (5) allergies; (6) autoimmune disorders; (7) degenerative problems; (8) accidents; (9) emotional disorders; and (10) a large group of idiopathic, unknown causes.

Many of the above categories actually describe pathological or physiological manifestations rather than precipitating causes of disease. Disorders of the "material" body are classified after the disease process has already effected specific tissue damage, because then the disorder is easily measured and categorized. The process that has occurred within the person himself, the underlying predisposition that allowed the disease to progress in the first place, is usually ignored. Questions that are overlooked include: What allows the bacteria, virus, or cancer cell to grow? What underlying factor is responsible for the system becoming so overly sensitized that allergies develop?

Concepts of Holistic Medicine

The therapies, philosophies, and medical systems incorporated into the field of holistic medicine are based on the actual promotion of health. They assert that disease originates *within* the individual. In accordance with this idea, in order for a medical system to properly be called holistic, there are six major principles which should be the basis of that system. These principles are by no means all-inclusive. They are, however, based upon clinical experience as well as philosophic consideration.

Mind-Body-Spirit Integration. A model of holistic medicine should recognize that the human being is multidimensional, not simply a physical entity that somehow develops a mind and intelligence as offshoots of the brain's physiochemistry. In orthodox Western medicine the split between the mind and body is reflected in the high degree of physician specialization. While specialists do great service because of their highly focused knowledge, they are limited in function and scope by seeing only a particular organ system and not the whole person. A typical example of this situation can be found in the headache patient who first goes to his internist. After his laboratory tests have been found to be negative, he is sent to a psychiatrist for evaluation. The psychiatrist probes into the patient's past, seeking something that may have predisposed him to headaches, but even after gaining some useful insights, the headaches remain. He is then referred to another specialist for further evaluation, but again the problem persists. What is missing is a unified approach that looks at the headache from many different levels simultaneously

Holistic medicine understands that man's total being includes the body, the breath (or energy), the conscious mind, the many levels of the unconscious and superconscious, and the spirit or Self. Because disease can occur on various levels, the holistic doctor must have approaches available that correspond to all of them. For example, if a person's breathing is characterized by jerks, pauses, or shallowness, and if in association with this he suffers nervousness, insomnia, and headaches, then it makes no sense to prescribe aspirin or valium. A holistic doctor sees the abnormality to be a breathing problem and teaches breathing exercises to eliminate irregularities, effecting a balance in the autonomic nervous system. (See Chapter 8, Stress Management Therapy.) The suffering patient thus learns to minimize his anxiety or headaches, as well as to recognize advance signals of distress and to prevent the onset of symptoms.

Self-Responsibility. As long as a patient blames the outside world for his ills, he remains dependent and avoids assuming responsibility for the state of his own health. He considers the weather, other people, or tiny microbes to be the cause of disease and feels that treatment should be directed at eliminating the external conditions or organisms. Holistic medical systems acknowledge that the environment is closely interconnected with human beings and may well contribute to ailments. Yet, as we have seen, they go further in maintaining that it is the inner state of the body, breath, mind, and habits that determine whether one is susceptible to illness. If he is balanced and living in harmony with respect to nutrition, breathing habits, and emotions, then external factors will have less affect on his general health. His immune system will respond appropriately to infectious agents and the nervous system will remain balanced.

What this means is that a holistic practitioner should help guide the individual to realize that he is responsible for his own well-being. Having recognized potentially harmful inner problems, the holistic doctor teaches the patient practical ways to change these habits and to replace them with positive, health-oriented ones.

Growth Orientation. An offshoot of self-responsibility is the area of the patient's personal growth. A holistic medical group should provide him with the stimulus and practical techniques for self-growth and enhanced knowledge. In order to guide the patient to new insights, the doctor or health professional should be a teacher as well as a healer. Once the patient becomes responsible for his own health care, he learns to expand his inner awareness of the obstacles that inhibit health. After observing for some time his own habits, modes of thoughts, emotional reactions, and how they affect his body and mind, he slowly gains greater control over them. Less energy is wasted in negative thinking which manifests as poor habits, abnormal breathing patterns, and overall body tension. As a consequence, more energy is conserved and is available to be channeled into creativity. Then, as his inner potential is gradually realized, growth and expansion of consciousness also occur.

Nonsuppression. In a holistic system the techniques for establishing physical and mental homeostasis, as well as the medicinal agents used, should not suppress symptoms. This can best be understood by using an analogy to psychotherapy. Thoughts and feelings that are repressed or suppressed are forced into deeper levels of the unconscious mind. Here they remain, causing the person either to act in unconscious ways, developing unconscious habits, or to erupt with uncontrolled and unpredictable force. In the psychotherapeutic process, the mental health practitioner helps the person uncover and re-evaluate this unconscious material and then to diffuse and channel the built-up emotions. (See the chapter on psychotherapy.)

Physical symptoms, similar to emotional ones, should not be forced deeper into the organism. It is generally not advisable to routinely suppress skin eruptions with topical creams, inhibit fever with antipyretics, or alleviate head-aches with aspirin. All of these symptoms are reflections of inner imbalances, and even if the symptoms are ameliorated by drugs, the underlying process that caused the symptoms to occur may still persist.

The therapeutic techniques of the holistic doctor are ones that lead to increased self-awareness and also strengthen the body's defenses. In the example of fever, the holistic doctor sees it as a positive signal that the body is actively at work defending itself. He may use natural herbs or homeopathic remedies which gently assist the body in the healing process and at the same time minimize the concurrent suffering. If drug or surgical intervention seems appropriate, the holistic practitioner will intelligently use these modalities. But after the crisis situation has ended, he commits himself to helping the patient quickly recover, and then he attempts to resolve the underlying imbalances which caused the illness. In essence, the holistic doctor respects the body's innate ability to cure itself and uses medicines which enhance that natural process.

Nontoxicity. Since approximately three million hospitalizations per year in America are due to the side ef-fects of drugs, the question of medicinal toxicity becomes quite relevant. The holistic doctor should study various sys-tems of medicine in order to determine the safest and most effective substances possible. He has at his disposal different remedies, herbs, and drugs, and he matches them carefully with individual problems and needs.

The idea of nontoxicity is the natural extension of nonsup-pression. The medicinal substances used by the holistic practitioner should not create more problems than the ailing person is already experiencing, and the medicine or the remedy should either help cure or palliate the symptoms.

Decreased Cost. Hospital costs and doctors' fees are exor-bitant and rising rapidly, and no way has been found to stem the inflation. The most feasible alternative is to remain healthy. A holistic system should teach people how to sleep, eat, breathe, and direct their emotions toward creativity,

The initial financial output in learning these things may be slightly more than the quick interview and physical examination that is often given. In the long run, however, the holistic system should save money for the patient and the community because one learns how to prevent illness before serious complications set in.

Conclusion

While the words *holistic medicine* have become popular in recent years, they should not be taken lightly. A doctor who calls himself holistic has a tremendous responsibility to both his patients and to society. Education, discipline, ingenuity, and a desire to integrate ideas from many areas are all essential ingredients for the holistic practitioner. The holistic patient has an equally important role in a holistic medical care system. He must be highly motivated, sincere, and willing to accept responsibility for his total health. Both physician and patient should look at all life circumstances as potentially growth promoting. Even illness can provide an opportunity for the patient to learn about himself. He learns to analyze the attitudes, fears, and habits that either precipitated or accompany his distress. The more knowledge and understanding he gains, the more aware he becomes. Slowly, inner awareness increases and as a result the doctor, the patient, and society become more whole.

11

Ancient Systems of Holistic Medicine

Both Eastern and Western cultures have developed schemes or patterns for understanding and describing man in terms of his physical, energy, mental, and emotional characteristics. In the East this organization of characteristics is seen as a direct reflection of the origin and order of the universe, or macrocosm. Man is seen to originate from within the universe; he is a microcosm or direct product of the greater order of the universe and as such is subject to its laws of interaction and transformation. Therefore, it is imperative that he learn to maintain inner harmony, or to re-establish this balance when lost, by following the laws of the universe.

Balance is the fundamental principle of order in the universe. This principle can be applied as a guide to all particular situations, including health; it is a basic law of nature which is expressed in the plant and animal kingdoms as well as in humans. Health is a state in which relative energy balance exists, while illness is an indication that this balance has been lost. This concept is fundamental to all medical systems, whether ancient or modern.

The ancient Eastern systems (Chinese medicine, Ayurveda, and yoga) acknowledge that accidents and climatic conditions, as well as bacteria, can create havoc. However, they also emphasize individual and societal responsibility for the maintenance of health. Common-sense preventive techniques are stressed, such as the healthiest way to eat, sleep, bathe, breathe, exercise, walk, evacuate, and have sex. Natural herbal preparations are the main medicinal agents of these ancient systems and are generally prescribed on the basis of specific symptoms and characteristics of the ailing individual.

3

Chinese Medicine

The Chinese approach to health maintenance and healing is but an extension of the basic philosophy that is reflected in all aspects of traditional Chinese culture. This philosophy, Taoism, stems from this ancient culture's concept of the origin of the universe. According to the oldest proposed theory of creation in Chinese culture, the three primary elements of the universe—force, form, and substance—were originally undifferentiated. In three separate stages, each one of these primary essences successively became distinct. At this point a separation took place: the light and pure substance rose above, producing the heavens, and the heavier and coarser substances sank down and produced the earth. Heaven and earth are differentiated through a harmonious, healthy, and dynamic balance. The maintenance of this balance is what is meant by Tao. Following the path of Tao, or maintaining harmony, means adhering to the course of the universe and adjusting to it. Stated simply, balance is the result of adhering to the laws of nature.[1] As in

---

[1]Huang, *The Yellow Emperor's Classic of Internal Medicine*, pp. 9-15.

the other ancient systems we shall discuss, it is evident that at the very foundation of Chinese medicine is a fundamental philosophy of existence that is laden with spiritual overtones.

Theory of Yin and Yang

In the original formless universe all imaginable things were totally merged in an indivisible unity. With the formation of heaven and earth, the universe was split and a duality was created—a duality that was totally integrated by virtue of its emergence from the same primordial energy of infinity. In Chinese cosmology this complementary duality of the two components of the universe, heaven and earth, is called yin and yang. The concept of yin and yang forms the ultimate principle of balance that is reflected in all phenomena. It is this dual power that is considered the initiator of all change. Change is the movement of one of the dual forces in relation to the other. Yin exists only in relation to yang and each gives rise to the other—as night begets day and day begets night. Yin eventually becomes yang and yang becomes yin as they are attracted to each other. Their relationship to each other and toward the whole is often illustrated by the concept of positive (+) and negative (-) poles of an electric current, each pole comprising a distinct but essential part of the same current.

Nothing is entirely yin nor yang, but everything contains proportions of both. Our internal and external environments are made of varying proportions of yin and yang. For example, our internal biochemical environment reflects the yin-yang composition of the food we eat. The relativity and pervasiveness of yin and yang are reflected in the yang quality of the surface of the body and the yin quality of the interior. However, even the interior of the body has organs that are made up of yang surfaces and yin interiors. Furthermore, the internal organs are made up of individual cells—each of which has a yang cell membrane and a yin cell interior. Thus, yin and yang are relative and not absolute, their relationship is dynamic, and their interplay produces growth, transformation and death.[2]

According to the literal translation of yin and yang, yin is the shady side of a hill and yang is the sunny side. But since yin and yang represent the ultimate principle that gives birth to all phenomena, their literal interpretation has been expanded to include all aspects of duality as reflected in the natural world: food, disease, the body, the mind, and morality. For example:

Yin	Yang
Female	Male
Earth and Moon	Heaven
Night	Day
Coldness	Fire and Heat
Centrifugal	Centripetal
Water	Dryness
Autumn/Winter	Spring/Summer
West/North	East/South
Interior of Body	Surface of Body
Solid Organs	Hollow Organs of Body
Sadness	Joy
Vice	Virtue
Disease	Health

Five-Element Theory

The five-element theory of Chinese medicine arises from the complementary duality and is the more tangible expression of yin and yang. Water, fire, metal, wood, and earth comprise the five primordial elements from which all things on earth are made. Man, being a reflection of the macro-

---

[2]Felix Mann, *Acupuncture*, p. 62.

cosm, is also composed of these five. These, of course, are not the same as the elements of modern chemistry. Rather, each element occupies a position on a continuum stretching from yin to yang: metal is the most yin, while fire is the most yang. Each element is associated with one hollow, yang organ and one solid, yin organ.

Among the five elements there exist certain relationships. The elements cannot only generate each other, but they can also destroy each other. Fire, or solar heat, animates the earth, earth produces the metals, metals (minerals) enrich the waters, the waters produce wood (vegetation), and wood gives rise to fire. This relationship is depicted by the outer circle of arrows in the accompanying diagram. Conversely, wood destroys the earth, as the roots of a tree penetrate the ground; earth inhibits water, as the banks of a river direct the stream; water extinguishes fire; fire melts metal; and metal destroys wood, as sharpened steel fell a tree. This relationship is represented by the inner circle of arrows in the figure. The balance between the nurturing and destructive interaction of the five elements is another reflection of the delicate balance of yin and yang.

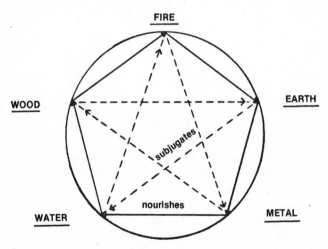

The Five Element Theory in Chinese Medicine

The Five Element Theory
in Chinese Medicine

In the treatment of disease, the laws that govern the relationships among the five elements can be used to correct imbalances of the five elements in the body in a reproducible and precise fashion. The interaction of the five elements infers that the body is not composed of individual organ systems that can be isolated and treated. For example, according to the five elements theory, treatment of the kidney will affect both the liver and the heart. The five element theory clearly highlights the idea of the unity of man and nature, a principle that surfaces in other holistic systems discussed in this book.

Chi As Energy

Ancient systems of medicine like the Chinese and Ayurvedic, due in part to the technical limitations of the time when they were developed, have placed less emphasis on trying to understand the specific details of anatomy, physiology, and biochemistry that modern medicine has extensively explored. The contribution of these older traditions has been in the direction of trying to understand the forces that animate man and coordinate his complex functioning. The Chinese call this force *Chi*, meaning Life Energy. Chi is made up of various components and is simply that quality which, when extracted from food, air, and water, animates life forms. Yin and yang are polarities of Chi. As the Chi energy enters the lungs directly from the air and indirectly from food and water via the stomach and spleen, it is distributed throughout the body in an orderly fashion through the acupuncture meridians. Chi is the power of enduring and continuing, or literally the vitality of the organism. Chi underlies mental, emotional, and physical health. It is similar to the prana of yoga and the vital force of homeopathy. Strengthening and redirecting this vitality is a fundamental goal in holistic healing systems, which all foster the principle of vitalism.

Acupuncture Meridians

The meridians are pathways for the uniform conduction of Chi to all the different hollow (yang) and solid (yin) organs. These are hard to correlate with any anatomical structure and many practitioners feel they are not physical but rather energy channels. However, Dr. Kim Bong Han of the University of Pyongang in North Korea, after extensive research and experimentation, believes that the meridians have a physical structure. According to Dr. Han, the meridians are 20 to 50 millimicrons in diameter, have a thin membranous wall, and are filled with a colorless fluid. At certain places, the channels send branches to the skin's surface, and these branch channels correlate with the acupuncture points. Besides the 26 principle meridians, there are numerous other energy pathways that make connections with virtually every cell of the body. These pathways are analogous to the *nadis* of yoga which carry prana to all body parts.[3]

The principle meridians are twenty-six in number—twelve of which are symmetrically paired on the limbs with one median meridian pair. The first three pairs of yin meridians are the heart, heart governor, and lungs and are located on the hidden, internal yin part of the upper limbs. The second three pairs of yin meridians includes the liver, spleen-pancreas, and kidneys and are located along the internal, hidden yin side of the lower limbs. The first three pairs of yang meridians are the small intestine, triple heater, and large intestine and are situated on the external yang

---

[3]Chang, *The Complete Book of Acupuncture*, p. 21.

portion of the upper extremities. The second three pairs of yang meridians consists of the gall bladder, stomach, and bladder, and they are located upon the external, yang part of the lower limbs and back. The paired median meridians are the vessel of conception and the governing vessel. The meridians affect not only the internal organs but also the various body parts associated with the internal organs. The body parts are associated with the various meridians, due in part to embryologic origins. For example, the ovary, uterus, fallopian tube, and testicle can be affected by stimulating the kidney meridian, since all these organs originate from the same embryologic tissue. Illness is associated with the blockage of energy in one or more of the meridians.

The Tao and the Cause of Disease

In Chinese philosophy the great middle path between the extremes, the Tao, is the principle from which harmony manifests itself. The theory of the origin of disease, as well as treatment, can be understood in light of this ultimate principle. It is taught that obedience to the laws of the universe is practiced when one has a modest life style and avoids excesses, while living with true devotion to others. To quote from *The Yellow Emperor's Classic of Internal Medicine*, . . . "those who disobey the laws of Heaven and Earth have a lifetime of calamities, while those who follow the laws remain free from dangerous illness."

The health and treatment of the spirit is indicative of the close connection between medicine and religion in Oriental thought. Currently in the West there is a reawakening regarding the importance of spiritual health as a prerequisite for mental and physical well-being. "Soul sickness" may eventually be universally known as a primary cause of disease. In Chinese medicine, treatment of the spirit consists of guiding the person towards the Tao, the unifying principle.

Persistent emotional extremes affect the Chi energy of a person. This is not much different from the modern model of psychosomatic medicine. Chinese medicine states that when one is excessively joyful, the spirit scatters and is no longer stored. Most people have experienced this as the "scattered" feeling of a fit of uncontrollable laughter. It is stated that excessive joy injures the heart, anger injures the liver, overconcentration injures the spleen, anxiety injures the lungs, fear injures the kidneys. It is interesting that the vertical wrinkle between the eyebrows which is indicative of liver dysfunction is easily produced by an angry frown!

Disease can also result from poor nutritional habits. As everything else in nature, food contains varying proportions of yin-ness and yang-ness. In order to maintain good health, the intake of yin and yang foods must be balanced. However, if this balance is not met, disease may ensue until balance of the diet is restored. The section on nutrition will expand upon Chinese nutritional philosophy.

The Chinese system of medicine, like all other holistic systems, is based on the principle that man's mental, emotional, and physical nature is part of a single continuum. In essence physical and emotional health are inseparable, and emotions naturally have an impact on physical health.

External Cause of Disease: The Weather and Heredity

Besides the "internal" causes of disease that have to do with spirit, mind, emotions, and habit, there are "external" environmental factors that are important in the Chinese concept of the cause of disease. Extremes of weather can injure the various elements and consequently the internal organs associated with that element. In a traditional medical practice, it is very easy to see seasonal patterns with arthritis, strep throat, skin problems, allergies, etc. In a similar way homeopathy pays exquisite attention to detail in its survey of the sick person's vitality, and every experienced homeopath is aware of how weather and temperature can precipitate many different diseases in people who are sen-

sitive to climate changes. Wind affects wood and can injure
the liver, cold affects water and can damage the kidneys,
dryness affects metal and injures the lungs, dampness affects
earth, and heat affects fire. The elements that are out of
balance are susceptible to injury by the weather which influences them. It then seems that the weather provides feedback on the stability of the elements. That is, if the elements
are imbalanced, the weather will bring this weakness to our
attention in the form of illnesses. Viewed this way, proper
treatment will strengthen that particular element and the
illness will subside as body balance is established. The
weather can be utilized as nature's way of giving a person
feedback about his relative state of element balance.

In addition to these "internal" and "external" factors that
are pivotal in the origin of disease is the concept of
hereditary predisposition. There are strengths and weaknesses in a person's genetic make-up that will be reflected in
his overall wellness. Included in this variable is the state of
the mother's health during pregnancy, for this will be
reflected in the health of the developing fetus.

Diagnosis

In Chinese medicine, the diagnosis is established after
gathering as much information as possible through: observation, interrogation, pulse diagnosis and palpation. The
technique of observation begins when the practitioner first
sees the patient. The information obtained depends upon
the sensitivity of the observer and his intuitive abilities.
From observation, the balance of yin and yang can be
assessed. Body structure, coloring, and personality characteristics indicate which element type predominates in a
person, shaping his physiognomy. The five human types of
Oriental physiognomy are as follows:

(1) Metal type, very yin: frail constitution, long face and

head, with the right shoulder often suppressed, long and delicate hands. These people are usually reserved, modest, and timid.

(2) Wood type, yin: long stature with wider shoulders. They are often patient, meticulous, and conscientious workers.

(3) Earth type, balanced: harmonious structure, precise gestures, good adaptability and flexibility, supple in action. They are usually calm and agreeable characters.

(4) Water type, yang: rather small structure, strong bone formation. They like good living, often become plump easily as they tend to be gourmands, and are easily attracted by all food that is yin, which tends to bloat them. Moreover, their tissues retain water easily. They are active, jovial, and full of good humor.

(5) Fire type, very yang: strong constitution, rather small structure, reddish complexion, small and thick, hot and reddish hands, well-developed musculature. Their trunk is very light, and they are usually proud, dynamic, and easily angered.[4]

The physician observes the mood, voice, gestures, and mental and spiritual aspirations of the patient. The breath odor and the condition of skin, hair, finger- and toenails will tell the trained observer much about the yin-yang balance of his patient. Knowledge of the qualities of stool and urine are necessary in terms of color, odor, consistency, etc. Similar characteristics of other body secretions are noted. Particular questioning will confirm or clarify evolving assessments of the yin or yang nature of the symptoms and add important information about past medical history and family health patterns. In this manner, a general picture of the physical, mental, and spiritual health of the person can be formed.

---

[4]Ohsawa, *Acupuncture and the Philosophy of the Far East*, Boston: Tao Books and Publications, 1973, pp. 27-28.

Feeling the pulses on the wrist areas is a means of monitoring the state of the blood and the energy circulation, and pulse diagnosis also provides information about the health of the internal organs. While in traditional Western medicine feeling the pulse is a diagnostic aid to help evaluate the status of the cardiovascular system, the pulse diagnosis is more elaborate in the Chinese and Ayurvedic systems. Six pulses are felt on each wrist. The physician lightly applies his first three fingers to the patient's wrist over the radial artery, which gives three pulses. Another three pulses are felt by each of the three fingers when applied more firmly to the artery. Many qualities of the pulse are noted—fast, slow, vast, weak, slippery, astringent, tight but thin, and tardy-irregular. Since each pulse is associated with a different internal organ, this aids in assessing the health of several organs. The pulses that are located on the right wrist of the male are located on the left wrist of the female and vice versa, yet another expression of the complementary opposites or yin-yang polarity.

The information about the yin-yang balance of the internal organs obtained from reading the pulses can be checked and verified by palpation of certain points located on their associated meridians in the abdominal area. Also, the bladder meridians that run down either side of the spinal column have specific pairs of points that are correlated to each one of the internal organs. They are known as associative points, and their palpation for tenderness will also check the accuracy of the pulse diagnosis. The path of the bladder meridian coincides with the location of the two principle nadis of yoga—*ida* and *pingala* (Chapter 5). In a similar anatomic distribution are the two sympathetic nerve chains of the autonomic nervous system.[5]

While similar to modern Western medicine in identifying the actual disease which effects the individual, the sophisticated Chinese approach to diagnosis is, more importantly,

---

[5]George Ohsawa, *Acupuncture*, pp. 27-36.

a means for assessing the strengths and weaknesses of each individual's vitality. Specific treatment modalities which strengthen the particular area of low vitality of the sick person are based upon this assessment.

Treatment

The methods of treatment utilized in Chinese medicine include:

(1) Curing the spirit
(2) Nourishing the body
(3) Medicinal treatment
(4) Breath treatment
(5) Acupuncture and moxibustion
(6) Physiotherapy

The discussion of spiritual treatment and nutrition was incorporated in the discussion of these factors as related to the origin of disease. *Medicinal treatment* consists of remedies of natural origin, primarily herbal in nature, knowledgeable application of which will assist in strengthening weakness and aid in restoring yin-yang balance. Medicinal substances are effective for they incorporate mixtures of the essences of heaven and earth, the basic substances, in balanced proportions.

Proper breathing is essential to maintain a perfect state of health and is necessary in correction of a disordered state. Breathing practices in Oriental therapeutics are quite similar to the pranayama techniques of yoga. It is mainly through the breath that Chi enters and energizes the body via meridian distribution. Yang respiration, which maintains energy in the lower, yang part of the body, promotes perfect health and is characterized by good abdominal respiration, utilizing the diaphragm. Breathing exercises in Oriental therapeutics are known to affect the internal organs, particularly in relation to the respiratory, digestive, and nervous systems.[6] Using electrical monitoring devices, it has been demonstrated that breathing exercises can affect and normalize the electromagnetic energy associated with the meridian points. The acupuncture points are the entrance points or "windows" into the meridians. It has been determined that these "windows" are better conductors of electricity than surrounding skin. Consequently, the specific acupuncture points can be scientifically located and verified. Breathing therapy balances meridian energy flow and increases electrical conduction at previously congested acupuncture points.

The techniques of *acupuncture*, *acupressure*, and *moxibustion* apply needle, pressure, or thermal (heat) stimulation respectively to meridian points to effect a change in the orderly flow of Chi through the meridians. This treatment helps to re-establish the yin-yang balance by initiating normal energy flow in stagnant meridians. The choice of meridian points to be stimulated is arrived at by using specific laws derived directly from the five-element theory and knowing the order of Chi distribution in the meridians. The five-element theory is the practical, tangible application of the complementary opposites—yin and yang.

The Chinese system of *physiotherapy*, or therapeutic exercises, is represented primarily in the practice of *T'ai Chi Ch'uan*, which is a system of exercises performed in close coordination with regulated breathing. The exercises are comprised of thirty-seven movement patterns, the composition of which is regulated by the principles of yin and yang. T'ai Chi Ch'uan will be further discussed in the chapter on movement therapy.

The therapeutic approach in Chinese medicine and all other holistic systems focuses on treatment which actually strengthens the person's vitality and raises his resistance to

---

[6]Palos, *The Chinese Art of Healing,* p. 152.

disease. Therapy may have its primary impact on a physical level through nutrition, or the effect may be mainly on an energy level as in acupuncture or breathing exercise. Lastly, the therapy may be directed toward the mental or emotional state of the person as in meditation. The ultimate result is similar in all cases in that all therapy strengthens the vitality that underlies the health of body, mind, and spirit.

Clinical Applications

As a theoretical model for conceptualizing health and disease, Chinese medicine helps to simplify understanding by highlighting the principle of balance. Maintaining a balanced vitality is fostered by an understanding of the extremes of imbalance, yin and yang. The concept of yin and yang is reflected throughout the natural world and provides us with the blueprints for understanding our own balance of yin and yang. Once this skill is mastered, the establishment and maintenance of a strong vitality is at hand.

The five-element theory and its application to the use of traditional Chinese acupuncture, as well as the complex system of pulse diagnosis, require years of study and application to master in order to effectively cure chronic disease. With less study, acupuncture or acupressure can be used to treat more localized problems such as stress-induced headaches or low back pain.

An aspect of Chinese medical therapeutics which requires less rigorous study, but which is extremely practical, is the concept of the different elemental types (metal, wood, earth, water, or fire). The ability to accurately recognize the various types leads to a greater ability to evaluate the yin-yang balance of the individual. This ability is fundamental to effective nutritional therapy. For example, a stout but muscularly developed man who generally displays an irritable temperament can be recognized as being of fire element, with a tendency to be overly yang. In general, he could be counseled to avoid too much salt and meat in his diet. This person would be classified as a mesomorph in Western terms, and the mesomorphic body type tends to have a higher incidence of high blood pressure and heart attacks. In fact, eating a meat-centered diet and excessive salt intake are risk factors for such diseases. Such a person with a predominance of the fire element would maintain a more balanced vitality by adding more fruits, vegetables, and whole grains to his diet. Similarly, a thin, pale, and frail person with bluish circles under the eyes would represent the metal type, which is an extremely yin vitality. In general, this person would be better off avoiding refined foods and excessive amounts of fruits and consume more whole grains, legumes, and vegetables.

Equally as practical as nutritional therapy in the prevention and treatment of disease is the use of abdominal or yang breathing practices. Chest or yin breathing is commonly associated with respiratory, neurological and abdominal disease. These diseases, as well as general anxiety or "stressed" states, are markedly improved by the establishment of an abdominal yang breathing pattern. These nutritional perspectives and approaches to proper patterns of breathing are the aspects of Chinese therapeutics which the authors routinely utilize and find extremely valuable tools in their own practices.

Conclusion

In summary, the Oriental system of medicine is another expression of the universality of the Oriental philosophy that applies to everything, conceptual or material. The forces that created the universe have a dynamic influence on all aspects of creation and are represented by the complementary opposites, yin and yang. Following this dynamic influence is the great middle path, the Tao—the path of harmony and balance. Straying from the middle path is ultimately the cause of all suffering and disease.

As in the other ancient systems which we will describe,

we see a strong flavor of a spiritual philosophy in Chinese medicine with an emphasis on the balance and unity that exists between man and nature. Chinese philosophy places strong emphasis on the vital nature of man and on the integration of mind, body, and spirit. Personal growth through expanded awareness is a direct result of following this medical practice, and this is a principle which is shared with other holistic systems.

4

Ayurveda

Originating in India, the medical science of Ayurveda has a very ancient and rich heritage. Although it can be traced back to the early Vedic writings several thousand years B.C., there is evidence that centuries before that a very sophisticated oral tradition flourished. Ancient texts claim that it goes back still further—even to the very beginnings of consciousness and life itself. It is written, in fact, that "there was never a time when Ayurveda did not exist," for every life form carried within itself the innate capacity to minister to its afflictions:

> The propounders of Ayurveda knew that the protective power and device was ingrained in life itself and acquired varied expression in the plant, animal, and man according to the exigencies that each of these states of animation gave rise to. The plant developed its thorns and a thick coat of bark to prevent its easy vulnerability. Animals and birds knew by instinct what particular action or thing helped to get over an affliction; and equally naturally did early man see with his mental eye the measures and things that relieved him of ailments. There was never a time when Ayurveda did not exist even as it was the case with life.

> The life stream carried in its current its own supporting
> and protecting wisdom that became manifest at the begin-
> ning of each cycle of the times of the seers. It is only in this
> sense the Ayurveda can be said to have a beginning.[1]

This is the tradition upon which Ayurveda is grounded,
according to the *Caraka*, a book which was written in approximately 300 A.D. and which still serves today as the standard medical text for aspiring students of this science. The
first section of the *Caraka* mythologizes the intuitive, self-
evident knowledge and universality of the principles of
Ayurveda. The *Caraka* also discloses the original intention
of its founders, which was to prolong the lifespan of people
so that the serenity and wisdom traditionally associated
with old age could become manifest. Hence, the literal Sanskrit translation of *Ayurveda* as "the science of longevity."

In those ancient times, there existed no sophisticated
technology or biological concepts to verify and scientifically
elucidate the laws of nature. All these sages had available to
them were the products of nature: herbs, plants, minerals,
animals, and themselves. They used their own bodies as
laboratories, and they were arduously trained in the skill of
self-observation. They devoted their lives to examining the
relationship between mind and body and how each was affected by the food they ate, the environment, and the subtle
impulses which surfaced from the deepest recesses of their
minds. Meditation was the technique that facilitated this
process, and by penetrating deeply into the interrelation-
ships between the senses, thoughts, feelings, and the
physical elements of their surroundings, these early healers
were able to extract the tenets upon which the science of
Ayurveda is based. Ayurveda is similar to Chinese medicine
in that it is based on a philosophy in which intuitive
knowledge provided a fundamental contribution to the
evolution of the system of healing.

---

[1]*Caraka Samhita*, Vol. 1, p. 38.

These observations of the order and nature of existence are as permanent and timeless as the universe itself, and so the principles of Ayurveda have remained unchanged for thousands of years. Ayurveda spread from the Himalayas outward to influence other cultures, including the Chinese, Persian, Hebrew, Egyptian, and ultimately the Greek schools of healing. However, it was in the subcontinent of India that Ayurveda made its strongest and most enduring impression.

According to Indian traditional teachings, life is not a finite experience demarcated by birth and death, but rather a continuous process with earthly existence and death as different sides of the same coin, much like waking and sleeping. During the wakefulness of life a person has the opportunity to grow, to explore, to evolve, and to look deeply within in order to come to an understanding of his underlying essential nature. It is also recognized that it is difficult to advance in perceptiveness when the body is ailing. It is not so much that illness is intrinsically bad, but rather that disease obstructs a person's ability to effectively perform his spiritual practices.

According to the *Caraka*, the primary reason for Ayurveda's existence was to provide the proper conditions for self-growth and evolution. It is in this light that a cure for man's ills were sought. Similar to yoga, Chinese medicine, and all other holistic systems, Ayurveda is founded on the principle of growth. In Ayurveda, knowledge of different health practices provides sound physical health, which sets the stage for spiritual growth. Ayurveda is not concerned with lengthening life simply for the purpose of increasing longevity, but rather to assist in increasing the depth and quality of one's existence. It is the duty of the Ayurvedic physician, or *Vaidya*, to provide the tools and to teach the proper habits, attitudes, and life style that will lead an individual to a healthy body, a clear, unfettered mind, and a reverence for his spiritual nature.

To understand the essence of Ayurvedic thought, it is necessary to let go of the limitations placed on reality by the present scientific models of the universe. In modern education the emphasis is on understanding the material nature of things. According to the tradition of Ayurveda, all phenomena, whether of a physical or psychic nature, emanate from one eternal, omnipresent, omniscient field. This reality, although capable of being experienced through higher levels of awareness, is inexpressible. By its unfolding, all else becomes manifest in time and space—every atom and molecule, as well as every thought and feeling. For the human being the physical body is the grossest manifestation, while more subtle human expression exists on a purely energy level. More refined still is the mental level, and beyond that still further exist even finer states of consciousness, the highest consisting of complete union with the original source, or universal consciousness. This theme of integration of mind, body, and spirit is identical to that of Chinese medicine, yoga, and all holistic systems of medicine.

The Scope of Ayurveda

The scope of topics explored in Ayurveda is vast. In the section of the *Caraka* on human embodiment, for example, varied subjects are discussed such as why the spirit, although all-pervasive, can be limited to local awareness in a human form. In the chapter which discusses conception and birth, there is also a treatise on the transmigration of souls. There are pages dedicated to fetal development, embryology, and the varieties and classifications of human body-types and psychological dispositions. These examples indicate that in Ayurveda the body, mind, and spirit are not compartmentalized, but that the three are interwoven in a subtle relationship, as intimate to the whole living being as are light and the eye to the perception of sight.

Other subjects included in the *Caraka* have to do with maintaining health and the prevention of disease. For example, the importance of dental care and oral hygiene are treated in detail, even giving directions on how to make a tongue scraper. It should be without a sharp edge and made from gold, silver, copper, tin, or brass. The teeth should also be thoroughly cleansed and the mouth washed to remove impurities which destroy appetite and cause diseases.

There are discussions on the regulation of sleep, hunger, thirst, and crying, along with warnings about some unhealthy practices, such as restraining the natural urge to urinate, expel gas, or evacuate the bowels.

A recurring theme running through the *Caraka*, as with the philosophy of the ancient Chinese, is that there should be moderation in all things. When contemplating changing one's habits, for example, a slow, gentle change is advised:

> By degrees the wise man should free himself from unwholesome habits; also by degrees should he develop wholesome habits. The acquisition of good new habits and the giving up of the old bad ones should be achieved by regular quarter steps of decrease as regards the bad habits and of increase as regards the good habits. By gradual withdrawal, addictions do not revert, and wholesome habits gradually acquired become firmly implanted.[2]

Finally, social responsibility as well as self-responsibility are stressed in Ayurveda. The *Caraka* enumerates codes of ethics describing the duties of the physician and the nurse as well as the responsibilities of the patient. Treatment of diseases and prevention of illness should be undertaken without regard for personal or material gain, solely for the welfare of the patient and the development of insight into the healing arts.

The Five Elements

To understand the philosophic perspective of Ayurveda in more pragmatic terms, we need to introduce the concept of the five elements. It is stated in the *Caraka* that all of what

---

[2]*Caraka Samhita*, Vol. 2, p. 44.

we call existence is composed of combinations of five basic elements: ether (space), air, earth, water, and fire.

It must be remembered that these elements are not in any way similar to the elements of modern physics and chemistry and Mendeleyev's Periodic Table. The five ancient elements represent a system for classifying phenomena. The element of fire, for instance, is not only associated with heat and flames, such as the sun, but is also the primary element involved with the digestion of food in the body and in the generation of body temperature. It is furthermore associated with anger, a short temper or choleric personality, various types of food, and is even characteristic of certain minerals and stones.

Tridosha

For the Ayurvedic physician, however, the five elements were not adequate for establishing a viable method of diagnosis, treatment, and prevention of disease. The system called *tridosha*, which incorporates the aspects of the elements but reduces the number of parameters from five to three, was therefore adopted. Tridosha refers to the three dynamic factors of *kaph*, *vat*, and *pit*. Each dosha or subtle quality underlies all existence, including the deepest layers of the mind, as well as the grossest body, sensations, and physical organs. Disease occurs when disharmony in a person's thoughts and habits disrupts the balance of the tridoshas.

Kaph is a combination of the elements of earth and water and refers to the qualities of solidity and heaviness. The word *pit* literally means fire, and this dosha is composed solely of the fire element. Whereas kaph tends to be cooling and unctuous, pit has the property of heat and volatility. Vat means "air" and is made up of the elements air and ether, and it is characterized by a light, subtle, buoyant quality. If one dosha becomes predominant, it drives the person towards illnesses that reflect the qualities of that dosha.

The tridosha system is strikingly similar to the five element theory in Chinese medicine and restates the principle of unity and balance that prevails between man's existence and the natural world that surrounds him. This balance and unity in nature is recognized as a basic concept in ancient medical models.

Ayurvedic Treatment

Ayurvedic treatment was the dominant form of medicine in India for several thousand years, but only in the last 200 years has the Ayurvedic physician come to share his responsibilities with the homeopathic and allopathic practitioners to some extent. Today, Ayurveda remains the primary treatment system in the villages where the availability of modern medicine is still quite limited.

In practice, Ayurveda encompasses a variety of therapeutic approaches. While dietary manipulation serves as a foundation for treatment, the Ayurvedic physician is also trained in other types of intervention. Often the approach used is designed for specific locales, as in the mountains of northern India. Here, where a great variety of different herbs are available because of the wide range of climatic conditions in the small geographic area, botanicals are used to a large extent. The ancient Vaidya, in fact, used a preparation made from a fungus to treat certain infections, as is done today in the case of penicillin. Furthermore, they had knowledge of the use of a potent drug used in the preparation of the antihypertensive drug *reserpine*, as well as many herbs to induce nausea, vomiting, or urination.

In southern India, with a lesser quality of botanicals available, more emphasis is placed on massage, bathing, and the use of emetics and enemas. Furthermore, the Vaidyas prepare medicines from minerals—some toxic in their native state, such as arsenic and mercury. Through proper preparation, the toxicity of the metal is removed, rendering a valuable therapeutic agent. It is interesting that some of the remedies take literally decades to prepare, and it

is the common practice for a physician to begin the preparation of a remedy so that his grandson can eventually use it.

Many other traditional Ayurvedic remedies and concepts
have found usage in modern medicine. Ancient medicinal
preparations are being scientifically analyzed in India today, and the results are quite promising. It has been recently discovered, for example, that both garlic and onions
prevent platelet aggregations and therefore may be effective
in preventing blood clots.

Noteworthy also is the degree of surgical sophistication in
Ayurveda, especially in the field of plastic surgery. The Indian physicians, using simple yet sophisticated equipment,
were not only able to sew back noses and ears severed in bat-
tle but showed a deftness that made them famous in their
own lifetime. It is only recently, with the advent of new
technology, that modern surgeons have been able to do
comparable work.

Clinical Applications and Nutrition

Some clinical applications of Ayurveda with respect to
diagnosis and treatment through nutrition can be found in
the sections on asthma, hyperthyroidism, ulcers, lower
bowel disorders, and skin eruptions and acne. A few specific
examples here will add greater clarity as to how Ayurvedic
principles are used in determining levels of health and
disease.

Ayurveda has interesting advantages over conventional
Western medical evaluation of disease. In orthodox diagnosis, there is no underlying principle that integrates mind and
body. There is no explanation, for instance, why a person
may be troubled with constipation, cracked nails, and fluctuating appetite, and at the same time has reoccurring
dreams of flying, insomnia, and is generally anxious and
fearful. A Western physician would pose several different
reasons for these problems and suggest many different drugs

and therapies. An Ayurvedic practitioner would perceive these problems as being related to an underlying predominance in the air element (vat). In this sense, Ayurvedic "physiology" transects the dichotomy of mind and body by showing that certain tendencies or ailments have their roots in an elemental imbalance which pervades both the physical and mental level. In this case, foods are prescribed that are low in the air quality and higher in the fire and water elements.

A concrete example is found in the case of diarrhea that occurs in the summer months. Because diarrhea is considered to be a fire (hot) ailment and because the summer is a hot season, then it follows that eating fire (hot) foods can further increase heat and cause diarrhea. The Ayurvedic practitioner would discourage the eating of hot foods, those which interact with the body to create heat. According to the Ayurvedic understanding, a food is hot because when it is ingested its chemical components induce secretion of digestive products of a particular composition appropriate to the food, and these in turn affect the endocrine system which governs digestion. Hormones are then secreted which produces the effect of the "heat" of the food by strengthening fire.[3]

In the above case, examples of hot foods are mangos and walnuts, while spicy food and cooking also increase the fire element. Cooling foods like yogurt and cooling drinks would be recommended to treat the diarrhea. By taking a preventive approach of avoiding fire foods during the summer months or by simply changing food choices if diarrhea does occur, the use of toxic drugs can be avoided.

Another example of the Ayurvedic tridosha idea can be verified by Western common sense. When a person has a mucus condition (kaph) such as an allergy or upper respira-

---

[3]R. E. Svoboda, *The Hidden Secret of Ayurveda*, Pune, India, 1980, pg. 17.

tory infection, seasoning food with cayenne pepper or ginger to make it hot (pit) will decrease the mucus-forming properties and clear out the sinuses.

Ayurveda also recognizes properties of foods in categories of dry or rough, oily or smooth, heavy or light. These properties also have therapeutic applications. Constipation is a dry condition (no water in the stool which is therefore hard or crumbling) and can be treated by oily foods such as coconut, fats, or ripe bananas. On the other hand, bananas that are not yet ripe would aggravate constipation and stop diarrhea. If a person had a runny nose, his discomfort could be helped by using more drying foods like millet, buckwheat, chickpea, honey, or black pepper.

Much of Ayurveda revolves around the medicinal use of foods and spices to prevent and treat illness. Related to this is the idea of taste which is expounded upon in Ayurveda. According to the science of Ayurvedic nutrition, taste is not only a function of a particular food but, more importantly, a function of the person eating the food. This can be easily verified by observing that when a person gets the flu, or in more extreme cases like hepatitis, food no longer tastes the same. Here, the food hasn't really changed but the eater has.

Another way to appreciate the idea of taste is by looking at how spices can be used. While Western science maintains that spices have little nutritional value and only add flavor, Ayurveda goes much further to maintain that spices also change a food's properties and affect the way the food interacts with the body. The subtle tastes of foods and spices have important affects on each of the doshas. The six tastes are bitter, astringent, pungent, salty, sour, and sweet. Honey is sweet according to this classification, but unlike most sweet food which enhances kaph and increases weight, honey is converted upon digestion to a pungent substance which stimulates fire (pit). Thus, honey in moderate amounts will not increase body fat but actually stimulates the body's heat and metabolism, dries up mucus, and can even help a person lose weight. Honey can also be added to yogurt—a mucus forming food (kaph) that can exacerbate allergies and colds—to decrease the yogurt's mucus-producing qualities.[4]

Ayurveda, based on personal experience of taste and reaction to food, is truly a holistic system in its relationship to nutrition. Food is seen to affect not only physical but also mental functioning. The principles of tridosha, properties of food, and taste qualities can all be used in a preventive and therapeutic manner.

Conclusion

For centuries, traditional healers throughout India have been applying Ayurveda to treat the sick. And although it traces its lineage to a period before recorded history, the timeless wisdom of Ayurveda is just as relevant and meaningful to modern man today.

As in Chinese medicine, Ayurveda is a complete system of medicine which is founded on both objective and intuitive knowledge. Ayurveda espouses a view of man which sees him as a part of the natural world and subject to the laws of balance that govern all aspects of nature. These laws are immutable and provide the blueprints for attaining the mental, emotional, and physical health which are necessary for ultimate spiritual evolution.

In the following section, we will examine the health practices of yoga science and philosophy, which were also developed to purify the body and mind to prepare the practitioner for the ultimate goal of spiritual growth and self-realization.

---

[4]R. M. Ballentine, *Diet and Nutrition*, pp. 437-439.

5

Yoga Science and Philosophy

Yoga philosophy asserts that human consciousness is multidimensional and that disease can manifest on any level of existence, ranging from the body to the depths of the mind. The "true" cause of illness, however, is believed to be within the subtlest layers of the unconscious mind. Misdirected desires that stem from the basic emotions and drives (sex, food, sleep, and self-protection) lead man from a state of equanimity and balance to disharmony, greed, and jealousy a state in which the external environment becomes something to possess, to conquer, and ultimately, to fear.

Desire, then, is considered to be the original cause of disease. As long as man experiences his unity with all things, he remains tranquil and healthy. This requires constant awareness that the inner self is one and the same as the universal Self. With such an awareness, one is fulfilled and his energy is directed only towards realization of this unity.

Yoga means union and stresses the integration of psyche and soma. Although this can be accomplished through several different paths within the overall system of yoga, raja yoga represents the most practical of the yogas in terms of holistic mind-body integration. It includes within its scope dimensions of all other yogic branches and systematizes them in a therapeutic fashion.

Raja Yoga

The codifier of raja yoga was Patanjali, a philosopher who lived well over a thousand years ago. There are eight steps in this system and each will subsequently be described. Special emphasis will be placed on how specific techniques associated with the eight categories can be therapeutically useful and how, by following these tenets, an individual can prevent illness and maximize creative potential.

The therapeutic implications of raja yoga are profound. The methods inherent to this system have been developed so that they slowly lead a person's body, breath, emotions, and mind to higher levels of refinement, alertness, and awareness. The eight steps are in a sense hierarchical, progressing from an individual's relationship to the external world and his interpersonal relationship to the deepest levels of internal awareness.

The first two steps of raja yoga are the *yamas* and the *niyamas*:

1. *Yamas* (restraints)
    (a) non-violence; not harming oneself or another, either by thought, word or action
    (b) truthfulness; not performing actions that are deceitful and not doing things that go against one's conscience. Untruthfulness can lead to inner guilt and has been associated with the development of disease.
    (c) non-stealing; freedom from thought or action colored by greed. Greed leads to self-indulgences such as overeating.
    (d) abstinence from sensual overindulgence

  (e) abstinence from hoarding one's own or coveting others' possessions
2. *Niyamas* (observances)
  (a) purity and cleanliness; of food, body, action and thought
  (b) contentment; learning to accept with a positive receptive attitude the fruits of one's actions
  (c) practices that lead to perfection of body, mind, and senses
  (d) study that leads to knowledge of the Self
  (e) surrender to the ultimate reality

These observances are essential prerequisites before beginning the more advanced practices of yoga. While seemingly simple in nature, each point has great depth and complexity. They help prepare and purify the practitioner's mind and body by stressing the mental and physical conservation of energy. Distracting negative and reactive emotionalism is discouraged. The yamas and niyamas "set the stage" for growth and internal observation by encouraging discipline, study, honesty, continence of speech and action, and contentment. Discipline need not connote rigidity or stoicism but, if understood correctly, can provide a channel for creative energy. Learning to be content in any situation eliminates the torment and obsessiveness that often lead to emotional or physical ailments. An attitude of receptivity and self-study enables the student of yoga to understand which habits and conditions inhibit wellness. Having gained such an awareness, he learns to avoid certain psychological conflicts, reinforcing instead those patterns or ideas which lead to psychosomatic balance.

The yamas and niyamas function as important therapeutic tools by preparing the way for the resolution and prevention of emotional problems, as well as for the expansion of consciousness. Self-observation and the elimination of dissipating habits are the foundation of health for the body, mind, and spirit. By observing the yamas and niyamas and leading a focused, directed, and moderate life, preventive medicine is practiced.

3. *Hatha yoga* is a system of various stretching exercises which when practiced are carefully synchronized with specific breathing techniques. Hatha yoga leads to greater health by reducing psychological and physical tension. (See Chapter 7, Movement Therapy, for further discussion of hatha yoga.)

The energy quality or the life force of man is described in yoga science as *prana*, which flows through various *nadis* or channels. Unlike the bronchial tubes which conduct air flow or the nerves that transmit electrochemical impulses, the nadis are not of material origin. They exist on a more subtle vibrational level and cannot be seen by even the most powerful electron microscope. They can be perceived only by constant practice of pranayama and meditation when the obstacles of bodily tension, breathing irregularities, and confusing thoughts are stilled.

4. *Pranayama* is a Sanskrit word which means the control of prana or energy through regulation of the breath. The breath is the main vehicle by which prana enters the system. By calming and directing the movement of the lungs, the person who practices yoga becomes aware of the existence of extremely subtle vibrations or prana. As he learns to use these forces, he begins to realize that the whole universe is composed of the very same subtle vibrations.

In the large sense, however, prana may also be considered as the fundamental Life-Breath of the universe. This manifests itself under five main categories or guises which are called in Hinduism *tattvas*. This refers to the mode of motion or impulse which keeps matter in a vibratory state. There are said to be five of these modifications of the fundamental Breath: akasha, vayu, tejas, apas, and prithivi, all of which in turn have their effects upon *Sthula* or the physical world. The five categories which apply at the psychophysiological level are *udana*, *samana*, *vijana*, *apana*, and *prana* (the latter, though with the same name, represents a subclassification). Each of these tattvas is associated with one of the five elements known to the Greeks: earth, water, air, fire, plus ether or akasha, the substrate of the rest. The body and mind, in turn, are composed of these elements of ether air, fire, water, and earth. Therefore, in this scheme, the tattvas nourish or strengthen both the body and mind of man.

Functions of the Pranas

Udana	Samana	Apana	Prana	Viyana
FUNCTION				
speech sensory separates body from mind	digestion metabolism assimilation	elimination excretion urination exhalation	inspiration	distribution and circulation of blood nervous system lymphatic system
LOCATION				
throat area	navel area	anal area	cardiac area	entire body

Pranic energy enters the body with the inspired air and immediately flows into the nadis located in the nose. Other portals of entry exist, and as one learns to follow the coursings, prana can be consciously drawn inwards at various locations such as the chakras, which are associated with areas of high concentrations of energy. (See Chapter 11 for more information on chakras.)

The number of nadis is approximately 72,000, and they are said to originate from the solar plexus center. Fourteen of these nadis are of importance, and when the nadis are concentrated in certain areas, such as the chakras, energy which is focused there strongly affects the individual. The flow of energy through the inspired air should be smooth and consistent because abnormal rhythms can create illness. Cycles of ebb and flow are established which correlate with normal physiological and emotional equilibrium.

Pingala is the first of the major nadis and it is associated with the right side of the body. It corresponds to active metabolic processes and sympathetic nervous system activity. Yogic symbology describes pingala as being the masculine, aggressive side, and its associated symbols are the sun and light. As air enters the right nostril, the prana is conveyed directly to the pingala located within the nose.

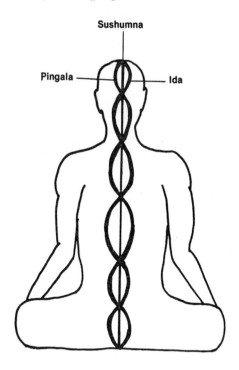

Ida is connected with the left nostril, the left side of the body, the parasympathetic nervous system, and the passive, receptive, dark, and feminine aspects of human nature. In yoga symbology, it is described as the moon.

Sushumna corresponds to the central axis of the body and represents the uniting and integration of pingala and ida. It is said to be located within the spinal canal of the physical body. Prana flows through the channel when both nostrils are directing the air flow evenly. The body and mind become calm and a meditative state ensues.

5. *Pratyahara* is the voluntary withdrawal of a person's senses from the external world. Health implies a keen balance between the outer world of sensory impressions and the inner world of silence. Techniques that help a person to screen out noise, sound, and sight enable him to be less affected by extraneous and superfluous influences and more confident and aware of his inner nature.

6. *Dharana* (concentration), 7. *Dhyana* (meditation), and 8. *Samadhi* (enlightenment) represent a continuum. In this system concentration is the focusing of consciousness on a single point; meditation is the sustained focus of a one-pointed mind; and samadhi is the absorption of consciousness with the object of concentration. The therapeutic use of meditative techniques will be discussed in Chapter 9, Psychotherapy, and Chapter 11, Yoga—A Complete Holistic Medical Model.

Clinical Applications

The preceding short discussion represents an overview of yoga as a philosophical system. In the later sections of the book, there will be a more detailed analysis of yoga as an integrating model that incorporates many other holistic systems. In these sections the therapeutic applications of yoga philosophy as a healing system will focus on the treatment of asthma, hyperthyroidism, ulcers, lower bowel diseases, and skin disorders.

Besides the diseases just mentioned, many other illnesses can be analyzed from the yoga perspectives. For example, in evaluating and treating headaches, a physician trained in yoga might promote changes in diet such as eating less stimulating foods (chocolate) and using more soothing or sattvic foods (vegetables and whole grains). The doctor might teach a cleansing technique like the nasal wash if sinus congestion seemed to be at the root of the headache. Breathing techniques such as the calming alternate nostril breathing might be taught, and specific facial massage and relaxing physical postures like the child's pose or corpse pose might be prescribed. (See Appendix for instructions on these techniques.) Specific visualizations, such as imagining blue light to permeate the painful head areas, might be prescribed to help relieve tension. Emotional problems such as suppressed anger might be allowed to surface during meditation, also to help dispel inner pressure.

Yoga as applied to health differs from Chinese medicine and Ayurveda in the sense that it is not a diagnostic system but a practical therapeutic system in which techniques can be used to maintain health, treat illness, and prevent disease. There are no real diagnostic methods such as the pulse taking found in Chinese medicine. There are no elaborate descriptions to analyze physiology. In a sense yoga is the therapeutic child of the parent system Ayurveda, specifically systematized for practical treatment purposes.

Yoga exemplifies the principles of holistic medicine discussed in Chapter 1. As a philosophic and treatment oriented system, yoga illustrates how the body, mind, and spirit are interconnected and interdependent. Raja Yoga represents an ethical system (yamas and niyamas with their focus on morals), a physical system (hatha with its many postures and cleansing techniques), an energy system (pranayama with its breathing practices), and a mental/spiritual system (pratyahara, dhyana and samadhi with focus on concentration and letting go of unnecessary desires). Yoga, is then, a system which develops the body, emotions, and mind so that they can be healthy vehicles to allow the inner spiritual and creative dimensions to unfold.

Yoga philosophy is vitalistic in that it acknowledges an inherent integrating energy (prana) that underlies both psyche and soma. The paradigm of yoga gives man a concrete way to bring philosophy and spirituality to the more mundane dimensions of health and illness. It promotes growth and exemplifies the unity of man and nature. Yoga philosophy supports the idea that by individuals attempting to better themselves and then teaching others various methods of health maintenance and disease prevention, the greater human community as a whole will benefit.

Conclusion

In spite of the many benefits of modern science, strict scientific models of the universe place restrictions on modern medicine. By contrast, ancient systems of medicine, born long before the scientific models were conceived, foster a particular reality of the world in general and medicine in particular. This reality goes beyond the strictly material nature which is the subject of scientific methodology. The ancient systems such as yoga blend intuitive and rational understanding to provide a basic foundation for relating to the universe. Man's spiritual nature is as important as, or even primary to, his mental and physical nature in these systems. The laws of nature are clear and immutable and indicate individual responsiblity and control over one's destiny. Health, happiness, and growth ensue if these laws are respected and followed; disease and unhappiness may fall upon those who choose to ignore them,

III

Modern Systems of Holistic Medicine

Yoga and the other ancient medical systems like Ayurveda and Chinese medicine have emerged in the Western world and are helping to free Western man from some of the limitations created by a narrowed focus on scientific technology. Studying ancient medicine offers us a fresh perspective on how to view our total nature: physical, mental, and spiritual. These philosophies contain the very seeds from which modern holistic medical systems have begun to grow.

6

Nutritional Therapy

The field of nutrition in holistic and preventive medicine incorporates knowledge from both ancient and modern medical systems and is one of the most important general areas. Achieving holistic health is virtually impossible with an inferior diet: malnourishment, due to deficient quality or poor selection of foods, often leads to physical and emotional problems. On the other hand, a diet which consists of natural, whole foods can lay the strong foundation necessary for health and well-being. Nutritious food supplies all the basic constituents and provides the fuel to sustain homeostasis of the mind and body, thus acting as a catalyst for inner growth.

The Importance of Nutrition

The necessity for good nutrition begins with conception. Thus, there is no more important time for good nutrition than during pregnancy. From the day a child is conceived by a poorly nourished mother, he is at a disadvantage. His growth is likely to be slower; he is more likely to be assaulted by infections and prenatal complications; and he is all too likely to be born prematurely, which exposes him to higher risks of brain damage. On the other hand, nutritional supplementation starting in pregnancy and continuing into early childhood creates more physically active children who demand much more of their parents' time and attention and who participate fully in the surrounding environment.[1]

Since the crucial period for brain growth occurs during the first six months of life, malnutrition after birth may cause irreversible brain damage. The earlier malnutrition occurs during this period, the more severe and permanent the effects. The impact of malnutrition on maturation can be so severe that irreversible physical effects occur and hospitalization for growth failure may be required before two years of age, or if extreme malnutrition lasts longer than four months during early life.[2] Mental effects of malnutrition in infancy are poor motivation, decreased attention, limited concentration ability, motor insufficiency, and retardation in sensory integration.

Beyond this initial period of brain development, malnutrition can significantly limit children's physical and mental abilities, as seen when children arrive at school without an adequate breakfast or if lunch is nutritionally inadequate. Hunger increases a child's nervousness, irritability, and lack of interest in learning. While there are no permanent effects on behavior or learning, hunger can disrupt the learning process because of inability to concentrate, which isolates the child.

Improper nutrition continues to effect a person's health adversely throughout his life. For example, there is clearly a relationship between inadequate nutrition and problems such as heart disease and cancer, the leading causes of death in the adult population.

---

[1]U.S. Department of Health, Education and Welfare, *Malnutrition, Learning, and Behavior*, p. 3.

[2]*Malnutrition, Learning, and Behavior*, p. 1.

Modern Nutrition

According to the modern science of nutrition, there are essentially five types of nutrients: protein, carbohydrates, fats, vitamins, and minerals. They are defined according to their biochemical structures and physiological functions. From the five basic nutrients, the body is able to manufacture all of the cells which comprise its structure (i.e., skin, bones, organs, etc.) and perform the functions necessary to maintain itself. These nutrients are utilized for such essential operations as growth, self-repair, production of substances necessary to guarantee reproduction (i.e., sperm and eggs), or protection of delicate membranes through mucus production. Some of these nutrients are converted into energy, which is necessary to power the entire process.

Western medicine has long recognized the importance of diet in physical ailments. High fat diets contribute to atherosclerosis, refined carbohydrates predispose to diabetes, and ulcers are aggravated by roughage and ameliorated by dairy and bland foods, and toxins from rancid peanuts may cause liver cancer. Vitamin and mineral deficiencies are also associated with physical illnesses, such as Vitamin A and acne, B_1 (thiamine) and beri-beri, Vitamin B_3 (niacin) and pellegra. Despite these contributions, modern clinical nutrition fails to provide adequate understanding of the subtler aspects of nutrition.

Beyond Modern Nutrition

It must be remembered though that food is more than just a combination of protein, fats, carbohydrates, and vitamins and minerals. We subjectively experience qualities or properties which are characteristic of each type of food stuff. Consumption of specific foods may affect individuals differently and in subtle ways. However, because modern scientific nutrition focuses on the biochemical and structural aspects of foodstuffs, many doctors are not educated in the medicinal properties of food or in the ways in which food affects individuals. It is taught that a balanced diet should consist of daily servings from the meat, dairy, grain, vegetable, and fruit groups for everyone, with minimal regard for individual needs. Meat and dairy are considered the most acceptable sources for complete protein. There is little emphasis on the need to eat fresh and locally grown foods. Doctors eat the same food and suffer from the same chronic degenerative diseases as do their patients.

In the past few years a few branches of Western medicine have begun to broaden the understanding of how nutrition can affect the emotions, personality, and mental states. Orthomolecular medicine and psychiatry have discovered that certain states of anxiety, depression, and schizophrenia may be due to vitamin and mineral imbalances. Foods that contain artificial colorings and preservatives can instigate hyperactivity in children and adults. Allergic reactions to some foods can lead to irritability and confusion.

When strict attention is paid to what is being put into the mouth, it becomes evident that each food not only has a different taste, smell, and consistency but also creates a unique subjective feeling. Eating a light salad leaves quite a different feeling from eating a big slice of roast beef. Eating an apple creates obviously different feelings in the stomach and mind than consuming a banana split. From the perspective of the Western scientist, these changes in the state of psychological functioning can be attributed to the pharmacological properties of food. Although food is primarily used for nutrients, many foods contain substances which have pharmacological effects on the mind and body. For example, milk and meat contain relatively high quantities of tryptophan, an amino acid that has a sedative property. This is one reason why a person feels sleepy after eating a large serving of meat or drinking a warm glass of milk at bedtime. Many other effects of food, however, cannot be as easily explained by simply using the laws of pharmacology.

By careful observation, it is possible to determine which foods create a positive effect and which a negative one. Certain foods, like grains and cooked vegetables, are conducive to feelings of calmness. Other foods such as fruits have a lighter or more energetic feeling associated with them. Some foods, like oatmeal, have a warming quality or a stick-to-the-ribs feeling. Others, like melons, create a cooling effect.

By paying attention to what foods in particular or what combinations of foods cause a bloated feeling, mental dullness, or emotional lability, a person can learn about his own particular reaction patterns and idiosyncracies. He can then intelligently alter his diet, eliminating problem foods and incorporating foods that lead to mental calmness and physical vigor. Coupled with a basic knowledge of nutritional requirements, a person can experiment with the subjective qualities of food and formulate an individual encyclopedia of knowledge based on direct experience.

Unfortunately, however, most Americans grow up on a diet saturated with sugar and chemical preservatives. They are accustomed to eating canned soups, frozen vegetables, and bread that stays "fresh" for weeks. The sense of taste and smell are dulled by cigarettes and air pollution. Eating on the run prevents any appreciation of the taste or consistency of food, much less its subtle psychological influences. Most people have lost the ability to discriminate for themselves which foods they really need to eat. The desire for food is based only on habit rather than the nutritional needs of the body.

The process of eating can be a means of self-expression and a vehicle for expanding awareness. What food an individual chooses reflects his attitude towards himself and the world. People who are always in a hurry will pick foods that are prepackaged, easy to prepare, and will frequent "fast-food restaurants." They eat quickly and may suffer from digestive discomfort such as heartburn, flatulence, diarrhea, and constipation. If a person is insensitive to his environment or to his inner feelings and urges, he will have little appreciation for the subtle tastes and smells in his diet.

However, anyone willing to make the effort, to let go of old habits and allow the intuitive senses to surface, will find that by merely assessing how he feels, the whole question of diet and nutrition becomes a simple matter.

Ancient Nutritional Therapy

Eastern traditions view man as a reflection of the universe, formed from the basic elements of the universe. Food also contains varying proportions of these elements and is needed to nourish the same elements in man. As explained concerning Ayurvedic practices, the ancients used their own bodies as laboratories, experimenting with different types of food to determine those best suited to their particular needs. From this experimentation evolved an empirical science of nutrition which revealed the most efficient ways to cultivate, prepare, and combine foods, as well as ways to use food medicinally. In other words, food itself, not just the extracted and concentrated vitamin and mineral fractions, is medicine. Nutrition forms the very foundation of health.

Chinese Medicine and Macrobiotics

Since man is a microcosm of the universe, ideally he is in balance with regard to yin and yang. Without the right yin-yang balance in the diet, the final construction and maintenance of each body cell will never be realized. Overeating in general or of a certain food group will affect the yin-yang balance and, consequently, the energy of the body. Whole foods that are in season and locally grown are ideal.

Cereals, especially brown rice, and vegetables are the most balanced in terms of yin-yang qualities. Thus, a balanced diet might consist of 50 percent cereals, 30 percent vegetables, and 20 percent from the other food groups.

Adding water or spices or refrigerating foods increases their yin qualities. Heat, salt (miso), aging, pressure, and dehydration increase the yang quality of foods. These factors that modify the yinness or yangness add a flexibility to this nutritional system. In hot (yang) weather, increases in the amount of yin foods (fruits) are acceptable to maintain balance. Indeed, in nature it is during the hot, yang summer that cooling fruits are plentiful. Conversely, it makes little sense to eat cooling tropical fruits in the winter for they will only increase coldness.

Yin/Yang Food Classification

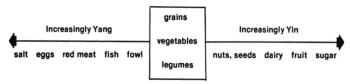

Nutrition, in a therapeutic sense, is very specifically applied in traditional Chinese medicine. The Chinese categorize food into five different flavors—pungent, sour, sweet, bitter, and salty—which have the effects, respectively, of dispersing, gathering, retarding, strengthening, and softening. These effects, however, exert their influence in relation to their associated element and corresponding internal organs:

> Metal .... Pungent .... Lungs
> Wood .... Sour .... Liver
> Earth .... Sweet .... Spleen
> Fire .... Bitter .... Heart
> Water .... Salt.......... Kidneys

Thus, the food, if chosen correctly, will help to supplement the function of the weak internal organ and related body parts. For example, if a person has a diseased organ associated with the element fire, he probably would be advised not to eat "bitter" foods as that quality is already overabundant. He might be told to eat foods that contain the flavor of "sourness" because of its association with the "wood" quality, which is believed to nourish or balance the fire element.

Ayurvedic Nutritional Therapy

In a particularly interesting section of the Ayurvedic medical text, the *Caraka*, diet and proper eating habits are discussed. An explanation is given of how to regulate the measure of food in proportion to the strength of the "gastric fire," or the body's capacity to digest what is put into it. Changes in diet should take into consideration physical constitution and exercise habits as well as digestive abilities. As in Chinese medicine, the type of diet to be recommended varies with the seasons of the year. Diet should be adjusted to the climate and the alternation of seasons, for as each season has a different physiologic effect, an appropriate dietary modification is required. The tridosha theory is applied to determine what foods should be eaten during which season. During the winter, for example, it is suggested that the diet consist mostly of heavier foods like grains and legumes, whereas the summer diet should be lighter, including more foods such as raw fruits and vegetables.

In terms of diet, heavy foods such as dairy products and meat are considered kaphic. People that demonstrate a kaphic constitution are large, often overweight, and tend to perspire easily. Kaph also implies the quality of psychological heaviness, as exemplified by laziness and apathy. In terms of eating, kaphic foods tend to make one feel heavy and lethargic and stimulate mucus production. After eating a very heavy and rich meal, a person often feels phlegmatic and torpid.

Physiologically, the seat of kaph is considered to be in the lungs and the upper stomach. Thus, in kaphic diseases like asthma and upper respiratory infections, there is often an increased production of mucus. Abstinence from kaphic food would be recommended to a patient with a cold who is producing a lot of mucus, to an overweight patient, or to someone who complains of lethargy and fatigue. Also, pittic foods that "burn off" kaph would be prescribed.

Pittic foods include peppers and other spicy foods. Pittic personalities are those intense, energetic, fiery, hot-blooded types. As one might expect in terms of the body, the duodenum and solar plexus are considered to be the location of the fiery element. Pit is that property that allows the body to burn food and transform it into energy. It is this essence which gives the gastric fire its power, and it is no wonder that a person who exemplifies a pittic personality, being easily angered and hot-tempered, often develops ulcers and stomach pain. The problem is that there is too much fire (pit), and he is actually burning himself up. The treatment would obviously be to reduce the fire by first cutting down on fuel, and then to cool it off with water. Thus the Ayurvedic physician would prescribe that the patient eliminate foods that create excessive quantities of pit, like hot or spicy foods, stimulants, and alcohol. Raw foods such as nuts and salads would also be eliminated because these foods are very complex structurally and require more digestive fire in order to be broken down. A suitable diet would consist of foods which have a cooling or kaphic effect, such as milk and yogurt, or foods such as vegetables and grains that have been well cooked. Cooked foods are more digestible and stimulate less pit to insure their assimilation.

Vattic foods are those such as fruits and raw vegetables. A vattic type of personality might be seen as intellectual, or light-headed and "spacy" in an extreme sense. Many mental disorders are often considered to be vattic in nature. Eating only raw fruits and vegetables tends to make one feel lighter and less "grounded." Too much vat can create an air of unreality, as well as lack of concern for others and irresponsibility. The center for vat is the colon, and many intestinal diseases such as diarrhea and constipation result from vattic imbalances. Vat is the energy principle that conveys motion, and its dynamic quality is apparent in the fact that constipation often leads to headaches. Vat, which normally moves downwards in the body, causing the expulsion of solid wastes, can on occasion move upwards. When this happens, the stool tends to remain in the intestines while vat moves upwards, manifesting itself as a disturbance in the head such as headache. Effective treatment for constipation is to drink a glass of hot water to which juice from half a lemon, a pinch of salt, and honey to taste, have been added. This traditional folk remedy is a very effective natural laxative and is very mild. It restores the normal movement of vat downwards, re-establishing elimination and allowing the headache to disappear.

Yoga and Nutritional Therapy

In yoga science, food is one of the vehicles through which prana is taken into the body. The physical, mental, and spiritual attributes of food are described by the gunas (rajas, tamas, and sattva), the three qualities of all manifestation. These qualities taught in yoga philosophy are comparable to the three doshas of Ayurveda and to the yin-yang theory of Chinese medicine.

In Ayurveda, stimulating foods such as spices are qualified as pittic. This stimulating quality of food is referred to as *rajasic* in yoga and yin in Chinese theory. Kaphic or yang foods, such as meat and dairy, which have a sedative effect, in yoga are categorized as *tamasic*. Those foods which are more balanced in yin-yang qualities (vegetables, legumes and grains) are considered to be *sattvic* in yoga. The right combination of fruits, vegetables, legumes, and grains helps to create a sattvic state of body and mind which is characterized by alertness and tranquility.

Each person has the ability to observe the effect that food is having on his state of mind. Irritability and lightheadedness are indications that too much rajasic food is being eaten: the qualities of lethargy and apathy result from an excess of tamasic foods. This knowledge of the subjective qualities produced in us by food increases the depth and scope of therapeutic nutrition, establishing nutrition as a major modality in the science of health.

Cultural Perspective of Nutrition

One of the first cultural and epidemiological researchers was a dentist named Weston Price, who in the 1920s traveled around the world studying health in various societies. Price focused on the number of dental cavities and deformities in facial structure in the population of folk cultures whose ethnic diets remained primitive and untampered with, as opposed to those of their relatives living in the cities. The latter were exposed to the influences of modern technology, including refined and processed foods. In every country studied, the people eating the ethnic, unprocessed diet had a far lower incidence in number of cavities, and also were less likely to develop the chronic diseases such as tuberculosis, arthritis, or diabetes that were beginning to ravage their city cousins. It made no difference, in general, what foods constituted the ethnic diet so long as they were locally grown and not tampered with. It was only when the native diets were abandoned in favor of canned foods, processed grains, and sugar, that health began to deteriorate.

Since Price's initial survey, there have been many other examples of people switching from their traditional diets to so-called modern ones, with the result of an increase in illness and a general decline in health. In South Africa, for example, despite the fact that sugar cane has been grown there for many years, it was only when the natives switched from their natural high fiber diet, which included raw sugar cane, to the more refined diet of their European counterpart, that the incidence of diabetes began to skyrocket. In Samoa and other Polynesian islands like Tahiti, the natives, popularized by Gaugin for their exquisite physical beauty and radiant health, now suffer from diabetes and tooth decay in almost epidemic proportions.[3]

In some cultures, it is common to find men and women living to be quite old. These cultures, such as the Hunzas in the Himalayas, the Russian peasants living in the Caucasus, or the Indians living in Ecuador, have received a good deal of notoriety recently. One common factor in all these people is that they tend to remain physically active throughout their lives. Secondly, and particularly relevant to this discussion, similarities exist in terms of dietary intake. Each of these cultures lives on a diet that consists primarily of grains—such as wheat, rice, corn—some form of beans or legumes, and fruits and vegetables. Meat is eaten only rarely. Again, the diet is devoid of processed or refined food and includes only naturally occurring, locally grown produce. Moreover, the agricultural methods practiced by these people indicate that they recognize the importance of keeping the soil balanced and fertile. Through terracing or similar procedures, erosion is kept to a minimum, and because of their proximity to the mountains, the water supply is rich in minerals. Thus, through cultural habits, these people have developed a harmonious and ecologically balanced system of food production. The end result is a culture nourished on natural foods, where longevity is the rule rather than the exception.

Nutrition in America

According to a government survey, which was done in 1965 to determine the quantity of different nutrients obtained in the average American diet, only 50% of the Americans were eating an adequate diet.[4] "Fat constitutes

---

[3]Weston A. Price, *Nutrition and Physical Degeneration*, (La Mesa, CA: Price-Pattenger, 1977).

[4]T. P. Labuza and A. Elizabeth Sloan, *Food for Thought* (Westport, CT: AVI Publishing, 1977), p. 150.

about 45% of the calories that most people take, and sugar accounts for about another 20%. Therefore, the diet of the average person is between 60% and 70% fat and sugar. Such a diet does not provide room for other needed nutrients.[5] Since World War II, the consumption of soft drinks has gone up 80%, pastries 70%, and potato chips 85%. Over the same period of time, the consumption of dairy products has gone down 21%, vegetables 23%, and fruit 25%.[6]

The 1977 Senate Select Committee report on the nutritional goals for the United States decided that there was a relationship between the current dietary habits of Americans and the incidence of cancer and heart disease, which are the two major causes of death in the U.S. The Committee advocated that people must return to a diet of whole grains, legumes, fresh fruits, and vegetables, supplemented by dairy and meat.[7]

Clinical Applications of Nutrition and Vegetarianism

With respect to individual, environmental, and population concerns, it seems reasonable for people to at least decrease their consumption of meat, if not to eliminate it altogether. The results of this could be improved health, more productive land use, and a more stable world community.

A shift in emphasis away from a meat-centered diet would be in agreement with the recommendations of the Senate Select Committee. The resultant diet would closely resemble that which is considered ideal by the Chinese, Ayurvedic, and Yogic nutritional systems. In addition, such a diet would closely parallel the type of diet chosen by

---

[5]Ballentine, *Diet and Nutrition*, p. 9.

[6]Lerza and Jacobson, eds., *Food for People, Not for Profit*. New York: Ballantine, 1975, p. 165.

[7]Committee on Nutrition and Human Needs, U.S. Senate, *Dietary Goals for the United States*, p. 1.

cultures which have proven to be superior in terms of health and longevity.

The advantages of vegetarianism include issues that relate to individual health, the bio-ecological balance, and the collective societal consciousness. The person who eats a meat-centered diet generally tends to overconsume protein and, as a result, the system must either eliminate the excess or store it as fat. High protein intake can predispose people to ailments such as gout and can be a burden on the kidneys. Vegetable protein sources usually have less fat than protein from flesh foods. Red meat has a minimum of 30% fat content, mostly embedded in the muscle tissue, even after the fatty edges have been cut off. Thus, atherosclerosis and obesity is less common among vegetarians and a diet based on whole grains and legumes can be recommended to those persons trying to avoid heart attacks or lose weight. If it is not possible to completely eliminate meat from the diet, it is wise to at least avoid excessive intake of red, fatty meats, using lean poultry and fish instead. This is preferable not only to lower fat intake, but because the carcinogenic chemicals such as nitrates in the food eaten by animals are concentrated in the fat.

From an ecological perspective, vegetarianism is a more economical alternative to serving the food requirements of the growing world population. For the same amount of usable protein, it takes ten times as much land to produce animal protein as vegetable protein. Cows require over twenty pounds of high quality, potentially human edible protein to produce one pound of animal meat protein. The industrialized countries, which contain approximately one third of the world's total population, feed their livestock approximately the same amount of high protein grains as the remaining developing countries consume directly as food.[8]

The term *vegetarianism* has several different connotations. Some people consider themselves vegetarians when

---

[8]Pfeiffer, *Mental and Elemental Nutrients*, pp. 106-108.

they abstain from red meat and eat only small amounts of fish and chicken. Those who avoid all flesh food, yet eat milk and eggs, are called lacto-ovo-vegetarians, and if they do not eat eggs, they are considered lacto-vegetarians. Vegans are people who eliminate eggs and milk as well as all flesh foods from their diet.

Many nutritionists are concerned that a vegan diet may lead to protein deficiency. These fears are based on the fact that abstaining from meat and other animal products (i.e., dairy) eliminates some of the best sources of protein. Inadequate intake of protein leads to symptoms of lethargy, weakness, depression, increased susceptibility to infection, and tissue and organ degeneration. However, a diet consisting of the proper combination of grains, legumes, fruits, and vegetables can provide a more than adequate supply of protein, surpassing the minimal daily requirement (MDR). It is important to realize that this MDR is a variable standard, dependent upon the age, activity level, overall health, and environmental situation of the individual. A general guideline is that for every forty calories taken in the diet, one gram of protein should be consumed. If an average diet is 2000 calories, then approximately 50 grams of protein would be indicated.

Protein is found in most foods in varying amounts. Some foods like dairy products, meat, or soybeans may contain thirty or forty per cent, whereas the protein content of fruits and vegetables is one to five per cent. Grains and vegetables are intermediary.

Proteins are composed of twenty-two amino acids, fourteen of which are synthesized in the body. The remaining eight are called essential amino acids because they need to be supplied externally through the diet. The amount of the protein eaten that is actually available to a person's body depends on the amino acid pattern in the food. The measure of biological value and digestibility is called the net protein utilization (NPU). The standard against which all other proteins are compared is the egg because it has the highest quality protein. In most other foods, one or more essential amino acids are absent or deficient, and these are called the limiting amino acids. The other animal products are closest to the egg in NPU—milk, fish, cheese, red meat, and poultry—and these are complete proteins. The vegetable proteins, including grains, nuts, seeds, and dried beans, are incomplete proteins because they lack an essential amino acid. Beans and grains are deficient in different amino acids, however, and thus when eaten in the same meal they complement each other and form a complete protein. Other combinations can augment the NPU, such as eating whole grains with dairy.

Modern scientific data supports the adequacy and even the superiority of a well-balanced vegetarian diet. For example, it is known that vegetarian Seventh Day Adventists have a lower incidence of high blood pressure, colon cancer, and heart disease than non-vegetarian Adventists or the population as a whole.[9] In the general population, blood pressure levels are higher in persons consuming food from animal sources.[10]

Conclusion

In holistic medicine, the trend is to re-evaluate the relationship between man and food and to observe the qualitative effects of food on consciousness. This careful observation of the subtle and gross properties of food with which ancient systems are concerned, combined with the contributions of modern clinical nutrition, provides the framework for nutritional therapy in modern holistic medicine. Defining the essence or the effects of each food as being yin or yang (Chinese), or vat, pit or kaph (Ayurveda),

---

[9]Armstrong, et al, *Blood Pressure in Seventh Day Adventists—Vegetarians*, American Journal of Epid 105:444-9, 1977.

[10]Sacks, Nosner, and Kass, *Blood Pressure in Vegetarians*, AMJ of Epid 100:390-398, 1974.

or tamasic, rajasic or sattvic (yoga), helps to create a workable model for establishing criteria to describe the properties of all foods. Combining foods according to these constructs, ensures a balanced diet.

Within this context, many people are now eating less fatty and heavy foods, such as red meat, and turning towards a diet which emphasizes natural, clean-burning, lighter foods such as fresh vegetables, fruits, legumes, and whole grains.

Nutrition highlights many of the principles of holism that ancient medical systems support. Good food nourishes the mind and emotions as clearly as it strengthens the body. Also, as people maintain a higher quality of nutrition, they become more conscious of the subjective effects of different foods, which thus expands their awareness and serves as a vehicle for growth. In addition, nutrition is a vitalistic science, as it strengthens resistance to disease by providing high quality "fuel" for increasing vitality. Further, the subject of nutrition deals with the holistic principles of balance and unity in nature as they influence the greater community welfare. Nutritional considerations force us to struggle to feed the animal life on the planet by using the most productive and ecologically safe means available so that all can share in the bounty which nature can potentially provide.

Principles of nutrition indicate the synergistic potential that exists between modern scientific knowledge and the intuitive wisdom of ancient systems. Modern clinical nutrition is in virtual agreement with basic nutritional concepts that have arisen in these less scientific and more intuitive systems. This is evidenced by the recommendations of the Senate Select Committee report on nutritional goals for the United States. There are many other important scientific verifications of subjective knowledge from ancient medical systems, which will be discussed in the chapter on the stress theory of disease. As a result of such discoveries, the future pursuit of knowledge in medicine hopefully one day may include the exploration of both subjective and objective information.

7

Movement Therapy

The Mind-Body Continuum

The concepts of "the body" and "the mind" are excellent examples of a dichotomy that is more apparent than real. Though words frequently give the illusion of a separateness and distinctiveness of the entity which they represent, that limitation often does not really exist. In actuality, the body and the mind can only be separated verbally; in function, they are intimately associated in the expression of the same person. Thoughts have a direct effect on the body. They are mirrored in the structure of the body as freely as the attitude of the body is reflected in thoughts and feelings. The exchange between the body and the mind is fluid and dynamic, the body representing the energy of the mind vibrating at a slower and more tangible frequency. Realization of the principle of unity that exists in this relationship between the mind and the body is fundamental to holistic medicine.

Yet, it is only recently that modern medicine has been able to accept this idea. From the time of Descartes until twenty years ago, medical dogma has embraced a dualistic concept regarding mind and body. According to Descartes, man has a mind and a body, but the two are separate and distinct entities. This dualistic attitude has been maintained in the mainstream of Western medicine. Modern medical research has emphasized isolating the particular bacteria or enzyme deficit as the important factor in a disease, whereas psychiatry has restricted itself to the analysis of emotional disturbances, often disregarding the general health of the body.

Specific Movement Therapies

The ancient medical and philosophical systems of China and India developed specific physical practices for identifying and then releasing tension in the body. It was observed that the physical body was the repository which stored mental and emotional stress in the form of muscular tension, glandular dysfunction, and nervous system overstimulation. The movements of T'ai Chi Ch'uan and hatha yoga were practiced to relieve this tension as it manifested on the physical level. The relief was experienced not only through improvement in physical health, but also, as elevated mental and emotional well-being.

Modern systems of therapy such as Reichian therapy, bioenergetics, and the sciences of manipulation also strive to balance a person's overall energy by working primarily with the physical expression of this energy. On the physical level, the neuromuscular system is the primary integrator of this process. The energy transformation that takes place on this nonverbal level can be co-ordinated with the energy transforming process that occurs on the verbal level in psychotherapy or other counseling. The energy transformed by either approach is the same, but a combination of the two methods affords more leverage to complete the process.

Hatha Yoga

According to yoga philosophy, health is the maintenance of balance or homeostasis. This state is achieved through the harmonious integration of the mind and body despite the internal turmoil precipitated by uncontrolled emotions and/or external environmental challenges. Every stimulus or challenge brings about a certain amount of mental and physical tension, and how this tension is integrated depends upon the stimulus strength as well as on the homeostatic ability of the mind and body.

The science of hatha yoga is a process of purification and strengthening of the physical body through the practice of various stretching postures that enable the body to become graceful, relaxed, and supple. Yoga philosophy explains that every mental disturbance alters the basic tone of muscles. Tone denotes the degree of contraction or tension of the muscles. Muscles can become chronically shortened due to excess tension, resulting in a shift in the underlying skeletal structure and manifesting as abnormal body posture. Besides the effect on the muscles, mental tension activates the endocrine glands and the autonomic nervous system (see section on Stress Management Therapy), resulting in overactivity of various internal organs, glands, and blood vessels. All these activations require energy to maintain, causing an excessive energy drain on the body, as well as limiting the body's reserves to cope with subsequent disturbances.

Correct psychological attitudes to minimize potential sources of mental disturbances is cultivated through observance of the yamas and niyamas. The practice of hatha yoga is important in helping to restructure abnormal body posture. It re-establishes normal muscle tone and flexibility that past mental disturbances have altered. This tone is a reflection of the psychological and physiological stability of a person and can be likened to the degree of tension of a bow. The effectiveness of the arrow that is launched depends upon the string tension. A loose string cannot supply force; an exceedingly taut string will have no recoil left to supply propulsion to the arrow. The arrow symbolically represents our ability to maintain or regain homeostasis or balance during stress. The homeostatic ability will be adequate only if the body tone is right, implying that psychophysiological balance exists.

Physiology of the Nervous System

According to Western physiology, the central nervous system consists of the brain and spinal cord itself. The spinal cord is lodged inside the spinal canal and is directly interconnected with the lowest part of the brain, the medulla oblongata. The cord begins at the first cervical vertebra directly under the brain and extends down to the second lumbar vertebra.

The spinal cord has several essential functions. Nerve fibers emanating from the cord form the thirty-one spinal nerves, which together with the nerves leaving the brain (called cranial nerves) form the peripheral nervous system, which spreads throughout the body. Within the spinal cord are important nerve fibers which are part of the central nervous system. They function to convey messages to and from the brain and the peripheral nerve branches, which is made possible via the ascending and descending nerve tracts. These tracts control most of our movements and many sensations: pain, gross touch, fine touch, pressure, temperature, and balance.

The spinal nerves emerging from the spinal cord activate the skeletal muscles by which we move our body. The sensory fibers of the spinal nerves receive stimuli from end organs of various types, such as eyes, stomach, etc. Each of these fibers conducts impulses toward the spinal cord from the particular receptor with which it is interconnected. Muscle tone is controled and monitored through nerve reflexes. The sensory nerve, which extends from the muscle to the spinal cord, measures the amount of muscle tone. This nerve then communicates with the motor nerve that extends from the spinal cord to the muscle fibers. The impulses that this motor nerve transmits stimulate contraction or relaxation of the muscle, which increases or decreases tone accordingly.

These reflexes are co-ordinated with other nerve reflexes which travel up the spinal cord to certain brain centers. At these brain centers the posture and muscle tone of all the muscles are monitored and adjusted to maintain the integrated structure of the whole body. These brain areas were the first to develop as the brain evolved, and they lie deep within the brain. They are referred to as the "lower" primitive brain centers and are controlled without our conscious direction. The reflexes that occur in the lower brain centers are modified by input from the conscious part of the brain, the cerebral cortex, which comprises the surface of the brain. The cortex is the latest part of the brain to evolve and is the "higher" center of the brain. It is highly developed only in primates.

The cerebral cortex control of primitive reflexes is demonstrated in patients who have suffered massive strokes with destruction of certain areas in the cerebral cortex. These patients involuntarily exhibit primitive posturing, such as rigid extension or flexing of their limbs. Ordinarily, the cerebral cortex has an inhibiting effect on these primitive postures, and when this inhibition is removed, primitive reflexes take over. Animals more primitive than apes do not have this conscious influence over postural reflexes, as damage to their cerebral cortex has no effect on their posture. These observations help to elucidate the neurological pathways which allow conscious thoughts and worries to affect body posture.

The Theory Behind Hatha Yoga

An objective in hatha yoga is to allow the primitive unconscious brain center to adjust muscle tone, unimpeded by inhibiting thoughts. This is done by assuming different postures or asanas, which leads to activation of certain reflexes which are integrated in the lower brain centers and normally function without conscious awareness. It is through these reflexes that normal muscle tone is re-established. The postures used are also primitive in that they mimic the positions of animals, as reflected in their names, such as the butterfly, cobra, and locust. Perhaps these postures facilitate a phylogenetic regression to man's evolutionary roots, where posture is not distorted by conflicts of the conscious mind. To ensure that the lower brain centers are free from the conscious cerebral cortical inhibitory control, the mind is focused on the breath. Free of the conscious influence, the lower centers may re-establish proper muscle tone through the adjusting reflexes initiated by the hatha postures. To summarize, mental disturbances can affect the tone of the body and upset the balance of energy to such an extent that normal homeostasis or body reserve is lost or decreased. By practicing asanas and concentrating the conscious mind on the breath, inhibitory thoughts and emotions can be released. Through appropriate reflexes, the lower brain centers adjust muscle tone.

The Theory of Nerve Reflexes in Hatha Yoga

There are thus several positive effects of this practice:

(1) Correct muscular tone is established.
(2) Energy wasted in maintaining abnormal muscular tone is released and can be used for more creative purposes.
(3) Distracting thoughts and emotions are rechanneled through breath awareness.

(4) Directed activity in the lower brain centers may help to liberate unconscious thoughts, memories, and conflicts which are stored in these centers. Release of these previously unconscious experiences allows them to be integrated into the conscious mind, resulting in expanded awareness.[1]

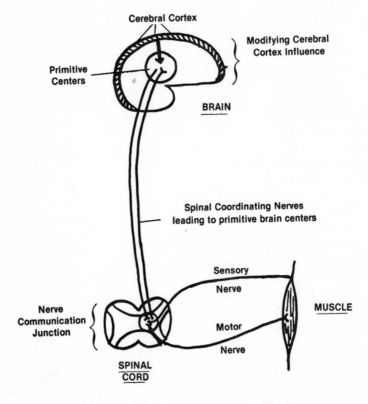

The Theory of Nerve Reflexes in Hatha Yoga

---

[1]Kuvalayananda and Vinesor, *Yogic Therapy*, pp. 20-30.

Nerve reflexes have further importance in understanding the beneficial effects of hatha yoga. Through nerve association, alteration in the tone of the voluntary skeletal muscles can be transmitted to the muscles of the internal organs. These reflexes are involved in some of the proposed theories on the mechanism of action of acupuncture and probably account, in part, for the efficacy of massage and manipulation. The theory is that embryologically similar segments of the body's musculature develop nerve connections along similar segments of the spinal cord. These connections are maintained throughout development up to maturity, even though some of the muscles are destined to become part of an inner organ system and others to make up the outer skeletal muscles. Because of this close connection or association in the spinal cord of nerves of embryologically related body muscle segments, stimulation of a nerve which innervates skeletal muscle may also excite a second nerve to a muscle of an internal organ. For example, embryologically, the heart muscle and arm muscles arise in the same body segment, and consequently their nerves are in close proximity to the spinal cord. Therefore, in the case of a heart attack where the irritation from damaged heart muscle is carried by the nerve to the spinal cord, adjacent nerves that normally bring sensation from the left arm may be excited. This explains the subjective feeling of pain in the arm which is a common complaint of the heart attack victim.

From a similar perspective, normalization of the tone of the skeletal muscles achieved in the asanas will also be transmitted to the muscles that line the internal organs, leading to healthier functioning of these organs. In order for these mechanisms to function optimally, unimpeded nerve outflow is essential. As the spinal column is strengthened and realigned through the practice of asanas, nerve pathways which may have been obstructed by distortions and deviations in the spine are now freed, insuring maximum efficiency in nerve outflow.

The Practice of Hatha Yoga

There are six *kriyas* or cleansings which may be used as preparation for the practice of hatha yoga. They are: *neti, trataka, kapalabhati, nauli, dhauti,* and *basti*. Neti, or the nasal wash, cleanses the nasal and sinus cavities (see Appendix). Trataka, or gazing, improves eyesight, cleanses the eyes, and improves concentration. Kapalabhati is a vigorous breathing exercise that flushes out the respiratory tract (see Appendix). Nauli is the separation and alternation of movements of the rectus abdominus muscles to aid digestion and bowel evacuation and also to stimulate the solar plexus area. Dhauti is performed by swallowing a strip of cloth to cleanse the stomach, esophagus, and throat. Basti is an advanced technique that is used to cleanse the lower bowel.

The manner in which an individual practices hatha yoga determines the quality of the benefits he will experience. A systematic program should be followed, allowing for gradual perfecting of the postures and incorporating the progressive development of the following qualities: flexibility, balance, strength, and stillness. In general, the beginner should endeavor to develop each of these qualities in that order, achieving a certain level of proficiency in each one before attempting the next. For example, initially the individual should practice gentle stretching exercises which are designed to increased flexibility and mobility of the body, thus laying the foundation for the development of balance. A stretch in one direction is balanced by a stretch in the opposite direction; any movement made with the right side must be complemented by a comparable movement with the left side. Only after the practitioner has attained a certain degree of flexibility and balance should he attempt the postures starting at the beginning level and concentrating on increasing flexibility and range of movement.

When working to increase flexibility, it is extremely important to establish a smooth, even rhythm to the flow of breath and to coordinate the breath with the movements.

Muscle tension creates blocks to the flow of energy or prana within the body, and also reflects psychological stress. Regulation of the breath helps to balance the autonomic nervous system and leads to a state of relaxation.

The release of muscular tension results in increased physical flexibility and also helps to liberate the pent-up emotions and conflicts that created the tension. In this sense, practicing the postures with some basic understanding of mind-body integration may lead a person to increased self-awareness. For example, the back is associated with active, aggressive "yang" qualities. Animals, when attacked, frequently curl up with the back exposed to provide defense. A person who experiences intense back muscle stiffness in forward bending may have overdeveloped defensive qualities in some aspect of his personality. Conversely, difficulty with backward bending may signify overly developed passive, protective, weak, "yin" qualities, which are associated with the undersurface of the body.

Understanding the subtle aspects of balance can also lead to important insights. Because balance and symmetry are continually stressed in the practice of the postures, differences between the right and left sides of the body become apparent: i.e., one side may be weaker, less flexible, etc. According to yoga philosophy, the right side is associated with aggressiveness and the sympathetic nervous system, and the left with passivity and the parasympathetic nervous system. On a physical level, the restoration of musculoskeletal balance leads to normalization of neurological function. Consequently, the equilibrium between the sympathetic and parasympathetic branches of the autonomic nervous system is maintained. As physical balance is restored through the practice of hatha yoga, psychoemotional equilibrium follows. It is in this sense that the system of hatha yoga can be employed therapeutically.

Only after the body has become more flexible and balanced should the individual attempt to sustain a posture for long. Holding a posture can lead to greater strength in the particular muscles involved, but strength is based on flexibility. If the muscles are still rigid and tense, trying to hold a posture will only stress the muscles more, causing pain and discomfort.

As the practitioner increases his capacity to hold a posture for extended lengths of time, not only physical strength but also mental and emotional endurance are enhanced. Most important, will power is strengthened. Any limitation which a person experiences, whether on a physical, emotional, or mental level, is the result of resistance. By progressively increasing the period of time a posture is held, an individual can learn to decrease his limits on a physical level and to cultivate the ability to work through and beyond the limits, leading to expansion. Working through or letting go of physical resistance can trigger a concomitant response on the emotional level, liberating the person from the subjective feeling of restriction.

Through the cultivation of self-discipline and will power, the practitioner becomes able to assume a posture effortlessly and to hold it without discomfort. Then the quality of stillness, in which all movement of the body and mind is quietened, can be achieved. The depth and degree of concentration and relaxation of the body is increased, and breath becomes very subtle. As a result, the practitioner lets go of body consciousness and establishes an awareness of the energy flow within. At this point, the mind can be allowed to flow with the breath; a mantra may be mentally repeated so that the mind, the breath, and the sound become one.

Though hatha yoga can be practiced purely for its physical benefits, the person who practices the postures over an extended period of time is aware that the real beauty of hatha yoga is its multidimensional process. The process involves a fluid, dynamic interplay between all levels of a person's being—body, breath, the various levels of the mind, and the spirit. This interplay reflects an equilibrium among the four qualities described above (flexibility, balance, strength, stillness). The advanced practitioner integrates all four qualities in the actual performance of the postures, thus fostering the development of these qualities in all levels of psychophysiological functioning.

T'ai Chi Ch'uan

The Chinese system of physiotherapy, T'ai Chi Ch'uan, is also a system of exercises performed in close co-ordination with regulated breathing. It has a similar effect on the mind-body as does hatha yoga. The exercises are comprised of thirty-seven movement patterns, the composition of which is regulated by the principles of yin and yang. The movements are slow, continuous, light, gentle, circular, rhythmic, energetic, graceful, and synchronized with inhalation and exhalation. In T'ai Chi Ch'uan the life energy, or chi, is built up and then directed, using the meridian pathways, to every part of the body to strengthen and energize every cell. The feet are firmly grounded and the spine and waist, or solar plexus area, form the sustaining pillar and axis respectively for the rhythmic movements of the rest of the body. This movement takes place under the concentrated, yet totally relaxed direction of the mind, constituting a meditation in action. As the student progresses in his practice and as his concentration increases, the movements become more subtle. Eventually, there is no movement and the chi is directed solely by consciousness. In the course of the exercises, virtually every muscle of the body is stretched and contracted, thus sharpening the sensitivity of the nervous and muscular systems. The overall effect is augmented physical, mental, and spiritual well-being, which help to build renewed health and contentment.[2]

---

[2]Edward Maisel, *T'ai Chi for Health* (New York: Delta, 1974), pp. 15-17,

The Mind-body Model in Modern Medicine

Modern medicine has also developed physiotherapeutic techniques, based on the principle of mind-body interaction. In the field of psychiatry, it was observed that mental conflicts tend to produce characteristic structuring of body posture. These observations led clinicians to question if correcting body structure would increase awareness of the psychological conflicts that may have led to imbalanced physical structure. One of these pioneers was Wilhelm Reich, a psychiatrist who proposed that the healthy and adaptable human being has an unobstructed flow of psycho-emotional energy which he called *orgone energy*. When there are mental conflicts, this normal energy flow is disturbed and increased in the form of psycho-emotional tension. Psycho-emotional balance is restored when this tension or extra energy is structured or stored in the body musculature. Reich attempted to reach and release this emotional energy through the integration of the physical technique of therapeutic touch with psychoanalysis, an unprecedented idea. His new therapeutic approach utilized the fluid nature of the mind-body relationship.

Alexander Lowen, a student of Reich's, has further explained this dynamic flow of energy between the mind and body from his own perspective. He calls the body's mental-emotional energy *bioenergy* and has refined a system of therapy called *Bioenergetics*. Muscular tension is seen as armour or a way to protection from feelings, desires, and sexual fears. A person isolates himself within a rigid shell of muscle stiffness. Underlying the body rigidity is the misdirected bioenergy which has become blocked in the physical structure of the muscular system. Various postures, breathing exercises, techniques of massage and manipulation, along with verbal expression help to redirect and realign this bioenergy. When it flows freely, the body and mind are again balanced and healthy.

Physiotherapy and the Mind-body Continuum

The techniques of manipulation and deep muscle massage also owe their effectiveness to the application of the mind-body relationship. We have seen that in Chinese medicine meridian points are stimulated to effect a change in the orderly flow of chi through the meridians. This treatment helps to re-establish the yin-yang balance by initiating normal energy flow in stagnant meridians, which leads to psychological well-being as well as physical health.

Massage has been used for centuries to help relieve physical and psychological problems. The reflex to rub injured parts of the body is universally noted, and today there are many different schools of massage which have developed and diversified this art. Massage helps stimulate muscular metabolism and increases blood circulation. It also stimulates acupressure points. Stimulation of other nerve receptors in the skin contributes to the general therapeutic effect of reducing physical and psychological tension and promoting relaxation.

Western healing systems have also developed manipulative techniques. Rolfing (structural integration) is based on the theory that emotional imbalances are projected outwardly as aberrations in structure. Thus, by restoring order in the physical structure, an increase in orderliness in psychological health is also achieved. This is effected through a form of deep muscle massage that attempts to free contracting attachments that form between the connective tissues envelopes that surround individual muscles. Without these hindering attachments, the musculo-skeletal system can assume a less restricted posture, often with the concomitant release or realization of feelings that contributed to the aberrant body structuring.

The traditional schools of manipulation, including osteopathy, chiropractic, and physical therapy, also release pathological body structuring through manipulation, often with marked psychological as well as physical improvement. Most illness, acute or chronic, has a musculo-skeletal component toward which the manipulative sciences direct their treatments. These treatments facilitate unimpeded nerve stimulation to body tissues by correcting nerve impingement at the spinal level. This results from abnormalities of body structure involving the spinal column and its surrounding muscles, ligaments, and connective tissue.

Aerobic Exercise and the Mind-body Continuum

Strenuous or active exercise also has an effect on the mind that may be due in part to its conditioning effect on skeletal muscles. Muscle contraction consists of two phases, isometric and isotonic. In the isometric contraction phase, the muscle contracts but does not produce any observable muscle shortening or movement. This phase is like a warming up phase, where the elastic components of the muscle are stretched before actual shortening occurs. In the isotonic phase, however, the opposite of the muscle actually move closer together, performing visible movement or work.

Active exercise improves the efficiency of muscles due to both increased muscle quantity or mass and nourishing blood flow. Consequently, less energy is wasted in the isometric phase that precedes the actual muscle shortening. For example, if you were not in good condition, you might waste hundreds of calories trying to pick up a 100 pound box of books and never move it. All of this energy would be spent in isometric contraction. In proper physical condition, the weight could be lifted quite easily, saving much energy. The conserved energy is then available to the organism for other uses, whether mental or physical. This explains the feeling of "lots of energy" from being in good physical condition.

Ayurveda extols the virtues of moderate exercise in which there is "perspiration, increased respiration and lightness of limbs," but condemns the evils of overexertion. Whereas the first leads to the "capacity for work, firmness, and tolerance to hardship," the second promotes "fatigue, exhaustion, asthma, thirst, hemothermia, dyspnea, cough, fever and vomiting." A person is truly wise, according to the *Caraka*, if he does not indulge in an excess of physical exercise, as well as inordinate "laughter, speaking, or the sex act."

Strenuous exercise also has an important eliminative function. Perspiration is increased; sluggishness of the bowels and of the circulatory and respiratory systems are reduced. Body fat, stored metabolic waste, and ingested chemicals are mobilized and excreted during active exercise. This eliminative effect is not only very important in specific therapeutic problems but is also psychologically uplifting. Exertion also increases blood circulation to many areas, including the brain. This increased supply of oxygen-enriched blood assures optimal brain function.

The number of people who are jogging is growing daily. People are rediscovering the joy of exploring their capabilities and endurance while running. They are finding that their limits far exceed their expectations. When the mind and body, coupled with the breath, are working together, the runner can focus his concentration and explore his physical and mental limits as he moves at different rhythms and speeds.

A daily program of vigorous walking, in which the movements are rhythmical and coordinated with the breath, can be enjoyed by those whose capacity does not allow them to run or jog. Walking can also be used therapeutically, as the steady contraction of all the muscles of the legs provides a gentle, continuous massage to the vascular system, thus increasing circulation through the muscles, relieving leg cramps, and reducing the tendency to varicose veins.

Recent studies have indicated that physical exertion also has a positive effect on the exerciser's eating habits. Exercisers tend to consume the same number of calories as nonexercisers despite the increased energy expenditure. Exercisers also, of their own choice, tend to consume foods lower in saturated fats and refined carbohydrates and naturally choose foods which are higher in vitamins and minerals. This is a fascinating and important effect of active exercise on mental functioning.[3]

Clinical Application of Movement Therapy

In choosing a suitable type of movement therapy, the needs and preferences of the individual are most helpful. If the primary goal is to maintain health and stay in good condition, then a good selection would be Hatha Yoga, T'ai Chi Ch'uan, or active exercise such as running, swimming, bicycling, or walking. Such active exercise may not appeal to some individuals or, as in the case of the elderly, it may not be desirable from a medical point of view. For such people Hatha Yoga, T'ai Chi Ch'uan or walking are preferable.

When selecting physiotherapy for the treatment of specific health problems, the degree to which physical or psychological symptoms predominate can be helpful. Therapies that have risen from schools of psychology such as Reichian therapy and Bioenergetics are more helpful when significant psychological problems which require ongoing counselling are present. On the other hand, for problems with a strong musculoskeletal component, rolfing, massage, or chiropractic are indicated because of the strong impact they have at the physical level. For example, chiropractic is very effective in treating acute and chronic musculoskeletal problems such as headache, backache, and sciatica which arise from accident, injury, overexertion, or stress. Manipulation can result in rapid improvement, and it should be coupled with advice regarding exercises to strengthen weak areas of the body to prevent relapse. For example, back pain which results from poor posture and lack of muscle tone due to inactivity will benefit greatly from practicing three sim-

---

[3]Cheraskin, "The Exercise Profile," *Journal of the American Geriatric Society*, Vol. 21, No. 5, pp. 208-215.

ple yoga asanas; the child's pose, the cobra, and the locust.
The Hatha Yoga asanas are quite effective tools for treating
many diseases because there are asanas to affect virtually
every part of the body. The shoulder stand, for example, is
very good for the thyroid gland; the plow stimulates the
adrenal glands; and the stomach lift is helpful for constipation.

Conclusion

A familiarity with the fluid nature of the interaction of
the mind and body is crucial for any individual who is
seeking health, growth, and freedom. With the exception of
good nutrition, nothing is more fundamental to establishing
and maintaining optimum health than some form of
exercise.

Movement therapies exemplify the unity of mind, body,
and spirit, as do the other holistic systems thus far reviewed.
Similar to these other systems, movement therapy cultivates
and maximizes individual growth as it helps to identify and
release the psychophysiological restrictions which limit and
undermine the vital nature of man.

8

Stress Management Therapy

The effects of stress, especially emotional traumas, and the relationship of stress to disease, have been known for a long time. The early Greek physicians recognized this, as did the early Arabic physicians. Avicenna, the most famous of the Persian physicians, established his fame by diagnosing love sickness and mental anguish in a woman who was without appetite, emaciated, and seriously ill. After being reunited with her beloved, she was cured completely. Ancient Ayurvedic physicians of India were also keenly aware of the indivisible reciprocal relationship between mind and body. It is stated in the *Caraka:* "The aggregate of the mind, body, and spirit is man,"[1] and also:

> The body and that which is called the mind are both connected to the abodes of disease. Likewise of well-being, the cause of which is their harmonious or concordant interaction.[2]

---

[1] *The Introduction to Caraka Samhita*, Vol. V., p. 4
[2] Ibid, p. 1.

Currently in general medicine practice it is generally observed that many illnesses are psychosomatic. This means that factors which lead to mental conflict eventually create imbalances in the body physiology. The altered physiology will, in time, effect changes in the tissues of the body. The tissue changes may result in tension in the muscles, ulcers, degeneration of the joints, or any other form of pathology. The psychosomatic theory of disease is clearly a reiteration of the holistic principle of mind/body unity.

Definition of Stress

Stress has been defined as a physical, mental, or emotional disruptive influence. Each person has his own personal definition of stress and has experienced symptoms of stress, such as anxiety, nervousness, rapid heart beat, cold and clammy hands, or muscle tension. Everyone knows what it feels like to be under strain, or to be chronically fatigued and "out of sorts." Indeed, for many people this state is the norm rather than the exception.

As scientists begin to unravel the mysteries of the brain and understand the relationship between the autonomic nervous system, the endocrine system, and the part of the brain controlling emotions and behavior, it is becoming increasingly clear that mental attitudes have a profound effect on physiological functioning. Stress, in the form of bright lights, loud noises, fearful thoughts, emotional trauma, and environmental or domestic pressures, can directly affect— via the autonomic nervous system and the neuroendocrine system—literally every cell in the body.

Physicians are beginning to see that the effects of chronic stress herald the development of a wide variety of diseases, ranging from the common cold to the classic psychosomatic diseases, such as hypertension, ulcers, and migraine headaches. More recently, stress has also been implicated as an etiologic agent in the onset of degenerative diseases such as arthritis, asthma, and cancer.

The Stress Response

To understand how stress is deleterious to health, it is first necessary to examine the basic nature of stress and the mind-body relationship. Over the millions of years of evolution human beings have developed a highly sensitive and efficient alarm system, and the primitive parts of man's brain are programmed to respond to stressful situations. However, modern living conditions have overburdened this sophisticated system. Civilization continues to develop at an accelerated rate and with such complexity that people are continuously exposed to high levels of emotional and physiological stress.

Under the surface of a supposedly rational twentieth century consciousness lies a less rational, more emotional, and very powerful, instinctual mind. Even if a person intellectually understands whether an event is serious or trivial, the instinctive or primitive mind may respond to a stimulus in the same manner as it has done over several thousand millenia, setting into motion the physiologic mechanism which can be identified as the stress response.

The stress response is the body's inherent mechanism for protection and, in this sense, is a vital and necessary adaptation for survival. The danger that initiates the stress reaction may come in the form of a natural disaster such as a fire, flood, or famine, or from the attack of a seemingly hostile person, animal, or bacteria. The stress response may also be a reaction to forces within a person's own system which have become destructive, as in the case of a cancerous cell. In all these instances, survival is dependent upon a quick and appropriate reaction by the organism. Pulling one's hand away from a fire, generating enough strength to beat off an attacker, or activating the immune system to increase the production of white blood cells and antibodies to destroy potentially virulent bacteria—all these are examples of healthy stress reactions.

Normally, confrontation with a stressor (the agent or factor initiating stress) is a "self-limited" experience because there is a finite time when a person is being attacked. Dr. Hans Selye, a foremost expert on stress, has called this response the GAS (General Adaptation Syndrome) and says it can be characterized by a specific set of physiological reactions. The GAS consists of three stages: alarm (or recognition), resistance (or dealing with the stressor), and exhaustion (or recovery, when the organism rests to recuperate from the trauma of the stress). This mechanism works well in cases of acute or "self-limited" stress. In the type of chronic stress that is commonly experienced every-day, crowded urban living for example, the third phase is never allowed to reach fruition. Rather than allowing time for rest and recovery from the exertion of stress, people become exhausted by a habituated stress response. As a result, they feel run-down and weak, with lowered stamina, and eventually resistance is lowered to a point where the organism becomes vulnerable to serious illnesses. The problem, then, is not stress itself but the prolonged or chronic stress response that lasts beyond the time that it is advantageous.

Stress and Disease

To understand the way in which stress influences the physical level, it is helpful to look at the stress response as it originates. The response is initiated in the brain, which interprets challenges as benign or threatening. The stress response is often consciously experienced as nervousness, anxiety, or fear. It would be difficult for a person to function if anxiety and fear could not be discharged and instead accumulated, interfering with the need for ongoing decision making. The tension generated by stressors has profound physical effects, so that in a sense, the body becomes a repository for psycho-emotional tension. The endocrine and autonomic nervous systems provide the avenues through which this tension moves via the brain to the body. Once stored in the body, this tension inhibits mental functioning, but to a less degree than its initial response. However, if this stored tension continues to accumulate and no means of release is provided, the body will reach the limits of its capability. At this point, the body itself may begin to break down, due to its inability to handle the steadily increasing burden.

The most outward indications of stress are the skin and the physical appearance. People suffering from stress often develop a washed-out appearance, with sunken eyes encircled by dark lines. Hair frequently falls out at an accelerated pace, worry wrinkles appear on the forehead, fists are clenched, and the toes curl under. Perspiration increases and constriction of blood capillaries causes cold and clammy hands—an obvious sign of anxiety.

Below the skin, the muscular system is encountered. Muscle tension is a classic sign of stress. At the end of a busy day, tight shoulders, tension headaches, "pains in the neck," and aching backs are all commonly experienced somatic symptoms of stress. In fact, certain forms of arthritis may also be secondary manifestations of the stress response. Constant tension in the ligaments and connective tissue around a joint may ultimately lead to an inflammatory reaction with pain and eventual scarring of the joint itself—all symptoms of clinical rheumatoid arthritis. It is not uncommon, in fact, for joint swelling to be preceded by nonspecific muscle or joint pain.

Moving further inward, the internal organs are also affected by stress. Tightness in the smooth muscles surrounding the capillaries and other blood vessels may occur, and if this constriction occurs in the coronary arteries, angina or myocardial infarction (heart attack) may be experienced because less blood and oxygen can flow through these narrowed passageways. Constriction along the arteries of the body can result in hypertension (high blood pressure), and if occurring along the cerebral arteries it may precipitate a stroke.

Increased gastric acidity leading to ulcers, chronic diarrhea, urinary frequency, palpitations, and wheezing are also related to stress in many cases, as are many sexual and reproductive dysfunctions, ranging from impotency and premature ejaculation in men to menstrual cramps and painful intercourse in women. Finally, and perhaps most destructively, stress has been demonstrated to influence the performance of the immune system negatively. Low white blood cell counts and thymus gland dysfunction have been observed in stress-induced rats.[3] Many researchers speculate that it is the deleterious effect of stress on the immune system that leads to a weakened resistance on the part of the organism, making it more susceptible to the development of serious diseases. It is well established that many chronic diseases including ulcerative colitis, multiple sclerosis, cancer, and the so-called auto-immune diseases are the result of a malfunctioning immune system.

The Physiology of Stress

The following information on anatomy and physiology is presented in some detail in order to help the reader understand that modern medicine corroborates ancient medical systems in the view that emotions and the body are interconnected. This background knowledge will be helpful in understanding later chapters, but it is not essential to memorize all the facts.

In general, the brain can be thought of as consisting of three parts which are arranged in a vertical hierarchy, with the more primitive functions being located in the lower parts of the brain and the more complex functions in the upper (higher) parts of the brain. The three parts of the brain are as follows: 1) cerebral cortex, 2) diencephalon or midbrain, and 3) medulla oblongata. As explained in Chapter 7, the lowest part of the brain, the medulla oblongata, is the

[3]Seyle, *The Stress of Life*. (New York: McGraw Hill, 1978) pp. 22-23.

most primitive part in terms of evolution, and its function is to control the most basic life support systems such as the heartbeat, respiration, and blood pressure.

Moving up from the medulla is the diencephalon or midbrain. In terms of the stress response, this is the most important part of the brain, for it is here that the instincts are mediated: It is through this part of the brain that the stress response is transmitted to the body. Located within the diencephalon is a part of the brain called the limbic system. Physiologists think that the limbic system serves as the "seat of the emotions."

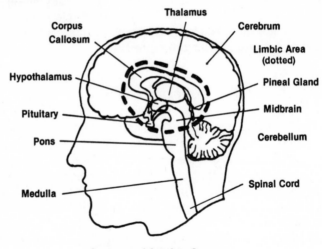

Brain and Limbic System

The highest center of the brain, the cerebral cortex, is located above the midbrain. As touched on earlier, it is responsible for the co-ordination of brain functions such as the ability to move, hear, see, talk, and reason. The information that is gathered here via the five senses is relayed to the midbrain and consciously experienced on an instinctual and emotional level via the limbic system. The limbic system can then send messages to the cerebral cortex so that emotions can be interpreted or "felt" via the higher brain areas. The cortex in turn can send inhibiting messages to the limbic system, protecting the person from reacting to every stimulus based totally on instinctive reflexes.

The limbic system also sends messages to the hypothalamus, a bean-sized organ located at the base of the midbrain. The hypothalamus controls many important physiologic functions, including body temperature, hunger, thirst, and sexual drive. Within its boundaries are the so-called pain and pleasure centers of the brain. Most important, the hypothalamus serves as one of the chief controllers of the autonomic nervous system and the endocrine system. The hypothalamus constitutes a primary regulatory center modulating endocrine and nervous system activity in response to messages it receives from the cerebral cortex and limbic systems. Thus, the hypothalamus provides the link to explain how thoughts (cerebral cortex) and feelings (limbic system) may affect the endocrine and autonomic nervous systems.

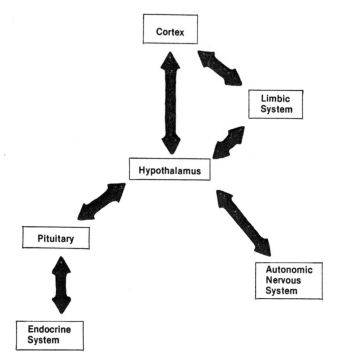

The Endocrine System

The pituitary gland sits right below the hypothalamus. It has been called the "master gland" because it releases hormones which ultimately control the activities of the other glandular organs within the body—the thyroid, adrenal, and reproductive glands. The pituitary gland receives messages from the hypothalamus either via direct neurological connections or through a special circulatory system between the hypothalamus and the pituitary. In response to these messages, the pituitary releases certain hormones which travel through the bloodstream to either the thyroid, adrenals, or gonads, stimulating the release of thyroid, adrenal, or sexual hormones respectively. Thus, a stressful thought originating in the cerebral cortex can directly affect the limbic system, which can then stimulate the hypothalamus and the pituitary gland, affecting the various glandular organs of the body. These glands have a profound influence on basic physiologic functioning. The thyroid, for example, controls metabolic activity, and if chronically activated via the stress mechanism, may result in rapid pulse, quick shallow breathing, sweating, and a general feeling of nervousness.

The adrenal glands are also very important in gearing up the body to deal with stressful situations. They secrete cortisone (a substance with anti-inflammatory properties) and other hormones which together regulate carbohydrate, mineral, and fluid balance. Chronic stress leads to overstimulation of the adrenal glands, which can result in carbohydrate imbalances such as hyperglycemia and a predisposition to diabetes and water retention. It is speculated, moreover, that chronic overstimulation of the adrenals may eventually weaken the body's capacity to fight off disease.

The adrenals also secrete chemicals that are intimately connected with the stress response. These secretions (adrenaline and noradrenaline) are compounds that serve very important functions in preparing the organism to deal with stress. Adrenaline causes mobilization of sugar from the liver by speeding up carbohydrate metabolism, providing increased energy for action. The pulse quickens, the blood pressure rises, and the body's arteries constrict to shunt blood to vital organs such as the heart and skeletal muscles, which need stimulation in order to sustain vigorous activity. The smooth muscles of the digestive tract are slowed down by adrenaline, thus preventing the digestive tract from using the large amounts of energy that are necessary to prepare for action.

The Autonomic Nervous System (ANS)

The autonomic or involuntary nervous system is that part of the nervous system which regulates the physiologic functions of the various internal organ systems such as respiration, pulse, blood pressure, reproductive functioning, and digestion. The word *autonomic* implies that these systems work automatically, without the necessity of conscious volition directing their functioning. This is in contrast to the musculo-skeletal or voluntary nervous system which regulates voluntary muscle movement. The arbitrary division of the two systems has become questionable since it can now be demonstrated through biofeedback that voluntary control of these so-called autonomic functions can be learned.

The autonomic nervous system has classically been divided into two interdependent subdivisions, the sympathetic and parasympathetic. The sympathetic system controls the functioning of active internal processes, and is the predominant system in dangerous situations. Activation of the sympathetic system induces the following reactions: pupil dilation, increased rate and strength of heart contractions, and constriction of the blood vessels that supply digestive organs and small muscles such as those in the hands and feet. Subjectively, these changes are experienced as feeling "bug-eyed," having a racing heart, and cold hands. All of these reactions are designed to prepare the body to deal with a potentially dangerous situation. It makes sense for the pupils to dilate so that a person can see better, for the heart to speed up to increase circulation, and for the blood vessels of the hands, feet, and digestive organs to constrict so that a larger flow of blood may be directed away from these less vital structures to the large skeletal muscles and the brain, which are more essential for dealing with an emergency. Other changes which occur during activation of the sympathetic system are that the hand, feet, shoulder, and neck muscles becomes tense, the throat tightens, and breathing changes from diaphragmatic to chest breathing, or the breath is held.

All of these symptoms, governed by the sympathetic system, are primitive instinctual reactions to danger. Problems arise, however, when these actions occur on a chronic basis because overactivation of the sympathetic nervous system can lead to the development of chronic states of disease, and ultimately to pathological illness.

Correction of this sympathetic overload depends, in part, on activating the ANS's other limb, the parasympathetic nervous system. The parasympathetic system can simply be viewed as the antagonist of the sympathetic system. Whereas the sympathetic causes constriction of the peripheral vessels, the parasympathetic elicits the opposite response of dilation. This is experienced as a feeling of warmth in the extremities, a slowing of the heart, stimulation of digestion, flushing of the skin, and a general sense of relaxation. In broad terms, the sympathetic activation is associated with stress and the so-called "fight or flight" response, while the parasympathetic is associated with relaxation and restoration of equilibrium. In actuality, however, it is not that simple. In certain functions such as sexual arousal, proper synchronization of both branches of the ANS is necessary. For example, in men the parasympathetic controls erections and the sympathetic controls ejaculation.

ANS Effects

ORGAN	SYMPATHETIC	PARASYMPATHETIC
Salivary gland	relax	secrete
Heart	accelerate	decelerate
Bronchial tubes	dilate (open up)	constrict
Stomach	relax (no secretion of fluids)	excite (secrete acid)
Intestines	retract	excite
Bladder	relax	contract
Blood vessels	constrict	dilate

Stress Mechanism

The stress-endocrine ANS mechanism may be simplified as follows: the cortex may send either inhibitory or stimulatory signals to the limbic system in response to a stressful situation. The limbic system in turn sends an emotionally colored message to the hypothalamus, which in turn affects the functioning of the pituitary gland and the ANS. For example, a person may receive a letter from the IRS stating that he is to be audited for the last five years. He reacts to this message by sending a message to the limbic system which evokes fear. The limbic system responds by signaling the hypothalamus, and, depending on how the hypothalamus has been programmed, certain messages will be sent to the ANS and the pituitary gland. These responses may be channeled through the hunger center causing "nervous" eating habits, or causing the hunger center to turn off entirely. The sexual center may be affected causing a decreased or increased production of the hormones which regulate gonadal functioning, resulting in decreased or increased sexual urges, again depending upon the way a person has been programmed to deal with stress. Aberrant functioning of the ANS may result in hyperactive bowels leading to diarrhea, or ulcers could appear as the result of a hypersecreting stomach.

It should be noted, however, that there need not be such a dramatic occurrence to evoke this kind of response. In people who have a low tolerance to stress, the same sort of response can occur from more subtle messages, such as minor disagreements with a business associate or spouse. While it is socially unacceptable to break into a rage over such minor disagreements, the primitive mind does not know this, and therefore the body's reaction may be nearly the same as in a more intensely stressful situation.

Finally, this stress response can be triggered on a chronic basis simply by some unconscious fear or fantasy. Many of the psychoanalytical theories which explain the development of ulcers, asthma, and other classic psychosomatic diseases speculate that the underlying cause of the disease is related to repressed fear that is expressing itself somatically. Often through psychoanalysis a patient may consciously contact the previously suppressed anxiety or fear and successfully reduce or eliminate both the fear and the symptoms.

The Stress Response and Individual Variability

The most important issues in the whole subject of stress are: (1) what constitutes stress, and (2) how can the response to stress be controlled. It is important to realize that stress is an internal phenomenon to some extent. This does not mean that external stressors do not exist, but people vary greatly in determining whether or not a situation is stressful. For some, traffic jams, preparations for a party, or overconcern about the welfare of their children are major sources of stress, while for others these situations are not stressful at all. It seems that a person's psycho-emotional balance may be crucial in determining how severe a disruptive challenge has to be before it is interpreted as stressful. An individual can learn to develop resilience, inner strength, balance, and adaptability so that the stress threshold is raised. This implies that his stress response becomes controllable: he does not overreact to challenges and his general reactive patterns to stress are appropriate to the stimulus.

There are challenges that would be stressful to the majority of people in the areas of job pressures, marital problems, financial difficulties, or the loss of a loved one. The intensity and duration of the stress response to these potentially disquieting influences is a reflection of a person's psycho-emotional development. Stressful situations cannot always be avoided, so the major goal in treatment is to prevent the stress response from becoming exaggerated or chronic. It is critical that the third stage of the stress response, the recovery phase, be allowed to reach fruition so that the neuro-endocrine and ANS do not remain activated.

The goal of biofeedback, autogenic training, diaphragmatic breathing, and all other holistic therapies that promote integration of the mind, body, and spirit is to raise the threshold to stress and teach control of the stress response. The concept of the autonomic system being "beyond conscious control" is now known to be a misconception; actually "involuntary" functions can be controlled by utilizing proper training techniques.

Stress and Biofeedback

As the the name implies, biofeedback is simply a way of "feeding back" to an individual information regarding a specific biological function. Just as the gas gauge lets the driver know how much fuel is in the tank, a biofeedback machine informs the subject of the level of muscular tension, skin temperature, or other physiological function that is occurring within his body. The machine translates this information into an audible sound, a flashing light, or some other easily recognizable signal.

The object of biofeedback training is to be able to consciously change the signal. When this is accomplished, there will be a corresponding change in the physiological function that is being monitored. To accomplish this, a new repertory of skills may have to be brought into awareness. For example, a person's finger may be connected to a bio-feedback machine which measures skin temperature, with the object of training as raising the skin temperature. This is helpful in many conditions such as migraine and high blood pressure. To do this, the subject must relax. This is because skin temperature is a function of the constriction or dilation of the small arteries in the hand: if the vessels are con-stricted, less blood will pass through and hands will feel cold. Constriction of these blood vessels is under the control of the sympathetic branch of the autonomic system and is a sign of stress. Warming of the hands occurs when a person can turn down the sympathetic hyperfunctioning. As this occurs, the blood vessels dilate, more blood flows into the hand, and the skin temperature warms up. This is indicated by a decreasing intensity of the audio signal on the feedback machine. Relaxation induces increasing hand temperature. Another way of saying this is that in warming the hands, a person is consciously reducing the body's stress response. It is through this type of biofeedback training, therefore, that a person can learn to gain some control over the autonomic nervous system and consequently decrease the stress activa-tion of the nervous system.

It is interesting that most subjects have difficulty per-forming such a task because they try so hard to relax that they actually make themselves more tense. They find them-selves competing against the machine instead of realizing that the machine is simply a mirror of themselves. The harder they try, the less successful they are, and often the temperature goes down instead of up, indicating that they are becoming more stressed. Eventually they get so frustrated that they quit trying, and at this moment an interesting thing happens. Once they give up or let go, the machine's audio signal slows down, indicating that the hands are warming up, which is indicative of relaxation.

Autogenic training uses the power of visualization in a positive direction and is helpful in normalizing the stress response. The thought of systematically creating a sense of relaxation, heaviness, and warmth in the body and mind will be transmitted from the cerebral cortex via the hypothalamus (and possibly via the limbic system) to the ANS to initiate relaxation.

Stress and Diaphragmatic Breathing

In the ancient scriptures it is said that the science of breath represents the vital link between the inner and outer worlds. Breathing is the only physiologic function that can be readily controlled by either conscious, wilful effort or by unconscious, automatic mechanisms. A man can choose to voluntarily alter the rate and rhythm of respiration, but if he is unaware of these processes, breathing continues on its own. This contrasts sharply with other organ systems such as the heart or digestive tract which function almost entirely on an involuntary basis in the average person.

The breath provides a bridge between the voluntary, consciously controllable, nervous system, on the one hand, and the involuntary system usually unavailable to conscious control, on the other. Thus, through breath control there can be some regulation of the autonomic nervous system. In addition, unconscious issues which often manifest as disturbances in the ANS may concurrently be influenced.

As explained in Chapter 3, according to Chinese medicine proper breathing is essential to maintain a perfect state of health and is necessary to correct a disordered state. It is mainly through the breath that Chi enters and energizes the body via meridian distribution. Yang respiration, or good abdominal respiration which utilizes the diaphragm, affects the internal organs, particularly in relation to the respiratory, digestive, and nervous systems.[4] Breathing therapy

---

[4]Palos, *The Chinese Art of Healing*, p. 152.

balances meridian energy flow and increases electrical conduction at previously congested acupuncture points, thus promoting health.[5]

In yoga philosophy, the actual mechanism by which mind and body interact can be more clearly understood through the concepts of prana, energy and breath. As described in Chapter 5, prana links the body and mind, and breathing is the physiological process most closely associated with this energy intake, dispersal, and balance.

Exercises which control and direct the breath flow help an individual to regulate the ANS, the emotions, and the mind, thus reducing the harmful effects of stress.

Shallow chest breathing is part of the alarm reaction and is associated with anxiety. Breathing with the chest physically stimulates the sympathetic nervous network that is located on either side of the spine in the chest area. Many people have adopted chest breathing patterns because they are subjected to heavy stress in daily urban living. Consequently, they experience a continuous state of low level anxiety which may be due to the abnormal breathing pattern. In chest breathing, there are many moving parts, including all twenty-four ribs and intercostal muscles; since it is difficult to synchronize all the moving parts, the breathing pattern tends to be uneven, which activates the sympathetic nervous system.

Conversely, learning to regulate the breathing patterns through diaphragmatic breathing can modify emotional states and restore equilibrium to the nervous system. Diaphragmatic breathing involves one moving part, the diaphragm, a thin muscle which separates the chest and abdominal cavities. Diaphragmatic breathing is smooth and has a calming effect, activating the parasympathetic system and resulting in an overall balance of the autonomic nervous system.

The practice of diaphragmatic breathing is basic to all other breathing exercises and is essential for the main-

---

[5]Ibid., p.76.

tenance of the health of mind and body. In inspiration the diaphragm contracts, flattens out, and moves down towards the abdominal area. This creates a large chest space and a negative pressure in the pleural cavity with respect to outside atmospheric pressure. The elastic lungs expand in response to this negative pressure. Air rushes inward through the nasal passages to the lungs, helping to equalize the different pressures. The abdominal muscles are concurrently pushed outward as the downward movements of the diaphragm compress the liver and spleen into the abdominal cavity.

During exhalation the diaphragm relaxes into a dome shape as it rises toward the chest cavity, squeezing the air out of the lungs. At the same time, the abdominal muscles move inward toward the back as the liver and spleen move with the diaphragm upward and out of the abdominal cavity.

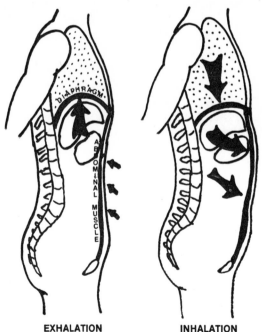

EXHALATION   **INHALATION**
Diaphragm Relaxes Upward   Diaphragm Contracts Downward

Generally, smooth diaphragmatic breathing is associated with good physical and emotional balance, while alterations and hesitations in the respiratory mechanism characterize disease. After an individual has found himself in a stressful situation or emotional crisis, a five-minute break of consciously performed diaphragmatic breathing while lying on the floor can help restore control. During the exercise, the mind is withdrawn from the troublesome issues and is focused on the rhythmical movement of the diaphragm, making it possible to view with greater clarity the source of feelings and confused thought patterns.

Learning to observe the breath's flow impartially creates a relaxed state of mind. During an actual crisis, breath awareness can help restore emotional and mental clarity. Muscle tension that went unnoticed before becomes apparent as the result of the relaxation that breathing exercises facilitate. Recognition of chronically abused areas of the body is the first step towards improving health. An asthmatic, by watching his breath, may learn that he holds his breath before the onset of an attack, and by adjusting the flow he may learn to prevent the ensuing bronchial spasm. A person suffering from ulcerative colitis may discover that he holds an inordinate amount of tension and blocked energy in his lower abdomen. By practicing techniques of breathing, he may learn to re-establish normal channels of release. Diaphragmatic breathing can be done while working with the biofeedback machine in a complementary fashion to demonstrate and verify its balancing or relaxing effect on the autonomic nervous system.

Clinical Applications

Because we live in a world permeated by high speed, constant change, and high expectations, stress reduction techniques can be useful to most people. Almost any disease—whether directly a result of high stress or because the illness itself causes stressful responses—can be benefited by stress reduction therapy. For example, diaphragmatic breathing is quite useful in such diverse problems as tension head-aches, eye strain, asthma, and ulcers. Breathing can help settle a person in the throes of an anxiety attack and can be used to regulate blood pressure. In the latter two cases, drugs and their inherent side effects can often be avoided.

Biofeedback oriented toward muscle relaxation (EMG) is useful in tension headaches, bruxism (jaw clenching), stiff neck, chronic back pain, hypertension, and arthritis. Skin temperature biofeedback in association with autogenic training helps such problems as hypertension, migraine headaches, and Raynaud's disease (cold hands and feet which turn blue or white, causing pain). EEG (brainwave) biofeedback has been used for insomnia, certain seizure disorders, and memory problems, and also to enhance more creative dimensions such as writing.

All these techniques require that the patient take the responsibility of practicing consistently and methodically. The self-growth techniques such as breathing, relaxation, or meditation will be only as effective and helpful as the energy put into them. This is true of all other holistic prac-tices. A person in therapy needs to work diligently to record his dreams and must have the courage to talk of painful feel-ings. A person under homeopathic treatment must learn to observe his symptoms and relate them to the physician clearly and concisely. A person prescribed a specific diet or exercise program will need to try to follow instructions closely to receive maximum benefit. It is only by trying and observing and adopting holistic practices that the patient can learn to discern his level of disease or health.

Conclusion

Essentially, then, the goal of biofeedback, autogenic training, diaphragmatic breathing, as well as other thera-peutic techniques used to counter the effects of chronic stress, is to induce relaxation within the organism and restore balance in the system. Whether this is a balance between the sympathetic and parasympathetic (which are terms used by Western scientists) or between ida and pingala (the two prime energy channels described in yoga anatomy) or between yin and yang, the basic underlying premise of restoration of balance remains identical.

Those who are unsuccessful in adapting to the requirements of life in the twentieth century are most likely to fall victim to the rash of stress-related disorders which have become so common in the last several decades. As a nation, the United States is in the throes of an epidemic of chronic degenerative diseases, and stress is considered to be a prime etiologic factor in the development of many of these. As the nature of living continues to accelerate in complexity, it is likely that daily life will become ever more stressful. As this occurs, learning to effectively relax and to maintain the physiological state of relaxation becomes not only a pleasurable experience, but, more important, a necessary survival skill. Just as the need to procure food and to procreate have always been conditions necessary to guarantee survival of the species, it now also appears that learning to maintain a mind-body in a relative state of relaxation is essential. It is not always possible to control external events, but each person has the capacity to control his inner environment. By assuming responsibility for the harmonious balance of the inner environment and by pursuing knowledge of alternate, more healthful modes of functioning, the challenge of this stressful way of life can be met.

This discussion of the stress theory of disease dramatically highlights the completeness of blending ancient medical philosophies with present scientific methodology. The ancient physicians' observations regarding the relationship of stress to disease can now be substantiated by modern neuroanatomy and physiology. This modern system maps out the details of mind and body integration, the fundamental principle of all the holistic systems. In addition, ancient medical systems provide useful tools such as breathing exercises and relaxation techniques which are invaluable in restoring physiological equilibrium.

This chapter and the two preceding ones point out three major areas of special concentration for holistic living: (1) nutrition, (2) exercise, and (3) self-regulation via breathing exercises and relaxation. Nutrition provides the building blocks of the body. Exercise reconditions the body, eliminates body wastes, and reduces mental tension. Self-regulation through proper breathing helps to reduce stress build-up, integrate the psyche and soma, and expand awareness. A person can appraise deficiencies and imbalances in this triad of health and then readjust his attitudes and practices accordingly. Nutrition, exercise, and self-regulation are the ABC's of healthful living and should be a fundamental part of every person's education.

9

Psychotherapy

Treatment of the suffering individual must ultimately focus on the mind, where, according to ancient medical systems, disease largely originates. Although Western psychology has played an integral role in elucidating human behavior, the split between man's psyche and soma has been widened by increased specialization in medicine and psychiatry. If the patient's problems are not viewed in totality, treatment can be fragmentary and the patient may not really understand how to interrelate emotional problems and specific physical ills.

Psychiatric inquiry and observation have described in great detail characteristics of emotional and personality disturbances. From a Freudian perspective, which is the prominent school of psychotherapy, underlying conflicts stemming from maladaptation in periods of infantile and childhood growth are analyzed in depth. Psychology, however, may be limited in scope in explaining certain aspects of human mental processes and behavior. There tends to be an emphasis on the negative, pathological side of man. Balanced health is primarily considered to be an avoidance of conflict and the maintenance of a "steady state" (ego) between inner needs (id) and outer demands (superego).

Prevention of mental diseases revolves around successful resolution of early infantile conflicts. Because of this disease orientation, the issues of growth and expansion are often neglected. Issues of man's potential creative abilities and positive expression of his inner self tend to be neglected, though Jungian psychology and some humanistic and transpersonal schools are growth-oriented.

Psychological study categorizes the manifestations of mind, the characteristics of personality, and qualities of emotional experience. It usually lacks a perspective of man's spiritual nature which is fundamental to psychological health, according to ancient medical systems. Questions left unanswered by psychological study are: What controls the mind? What are the underlying causes of emotion? What are thoughts and how can they be positively directed and controlled? What are the different levels of the unconscious? How does man's individual consciousness fit into the universal consciousness?

Abraham Maslow and Roberto Assagioli have attempted to explain the underlying nature of psychological health, the experiences which are common to individuals who maximize their creative and intellectual abilities, along with various techniques useful in the quest for inner knowledge, wisdom, and fulfillment. These conceptualizations are colloquially called the Third Force, or humanistic or transcendental psychology. In this context, the first force is behavioral psychology which encompasses the objective and more mechanistic theories of human behavior. The second force is composed of the various schools of psychology that originated from Freud and psychoanalysis, which include: psychosomatic medicine, Freudian psychoanalysis, Jungian analytical psychology, and Gestalt Therapy.

The First Force: Behavioral Psychology

From the perspective of behavioral psychology, a person's reactions and emotional character directly reflect the positive or negative rewards or punishments he receives. For instance, the therapist might have a patient push a hand-held digital counter each time he bites his nails. If praise is given in response to a certain action, then that action is rein-forced and later repeated. Behaviorism, in a general sense, represents a conditioning process. A behavior therapist might teach relaxation techniques or promote positive habits to substitute for habits that interfere with a person's well-being.

The Second Force: Psychosomatic Medicine, Freudian and Jungian Psychologies

Psychosomatic medicine, an offshoot of classical Freudian psychology, was systematized by Franz Alexander in the 1940s. While recognizing that emotional problems are re-lated to internal conflicts, defenses, and repressed feelings, psychosomatic medicine attempts to explain how these af-fect specific body parts and cause certain physical diseases. Thus, psychosomatic medicine attempts to bridge the gap between mind and body. This model represents a prominent Western approach to holism through the synthesis of psy-chology and medicine. The appreciation of the interconnec-tions between the dynamics of mental processes and the body's physiology leads to a greater understanding of the integrated nature of the human being.

Classical medicine has defined the term *psychosomatic* to imply specific illnesses which could be described by their pathological changes, but which also seemed to be linked to a disturbed emotional state. For example, peptic ulcer dis-ease, rheumatoid arthritis, asthma, and ulcerative colitis are classic psychosomatic diseases. Subsequently, the term *psychosomatic* has been redefined and used colloquially to include those diseases for which no biochemical or X-ray abnormality can be found but which still lead the patient to seek medical aid. Thus, many types of chest, stomach, and back pains, as well as complaints of numbness or ringing in the ears, which are enigmas in conventional diagnosis, are now labeled "psychosomatic."

This latter usage of the term *psychosomatic disorders* is not the concept being defined in this section. Psychosomatic medicine is a distinct field of inquiry which uses psychological techniques and language to describe the linkage between emotions and physiology. This system incorporates psychoanalytical methodology to interpret how psychological conflict affects physical functioning as projected through the autonomic nervous system. Thus far, only a few specific diseases have been identified as being classically psychosomatic. As further scientific and psychiatric research continues, many more illnesses will probably be included in the field of psychosomatic medicine. By combining holistic medical perspectives and the knowledge of ancient medical systems with modern medical theory and technology, mental and physical processes may be seen to be truly inseparable, and the practice of classifying disease as physical or mental may become obsolete. To say that a disease is "only in the patient's mind" is to erroneously minimize the importance of the direct effect that thoughts and feelings have on body physiology. We can only speculate on the reason that some people react to emotional conflict and develop disease, while other people who are subjected to similar situations remain free of illness. Those who develop actual disease are in some way unable to adapt to the various problems that arise during life. They cannot "let go" of certain patterns of response and this leads to physical illness.

Expression of Psychological Conflict. According to psychosomatic medicine, psychological conflicts can influence a person's physiology in a number of ways. There may be a modification of (1) satisfaction of basic needs, (2) emotional expression, and (3) nervous system activity.

Psychological imbalances can affect the voluntary activities which deal with the satisfaction of primary needs such as hunger, self-protection, sleep, and sex. A person generally has voluntary control of when and how to satisfy these basic needs. Suppressed emotional conflicts can cause distortion or loss of this control, resulting in physical discomfort or disease. The malady anorexia nervosa exemplifies this problem. A person exhibiting symptoms of this disorder experiences complete loss of appetite, perhaps as a result of chronic depression or unresolved anger. This leads to the obvious physical problem of malnutrition.

Psychological conflicts may affect the means of emotional self-expression such as laughing, crying, or blushing. When these conflicts are repressed, certain physical problems arise. For example, suppression of anxiety may lead to an inappropriate affect such as hysterical, uncontrolled laughter. Also, if a person's feelings are inhibited, abnormal body posturing or tics may result. If maintained over a prolonged period of time, irregularities in posture can lead to structural deviation in the musculoskeletal system, resulting in such problems as chronic arthritis.

Psychological factors also affect the autonomic nervous system and the physiological functions under its control. It is here that psychosomatic medicine focuses most of its attention. In this context, psychosomatic medicine is concerned with specific illnesses or physiological processes which have psychological counterparts, perceived subjectively as emotions and desires.

Psychosomatic Medicine and the Autonomic Nervous System. Activation of the sympathetic system is associated with *active* responses (physical or emotional) in general, and activation of the parasympathetic nervous system is associated with *passive* responses (physical or emotional) in general. According to psychosomatic medicine, a person may respond actively to conflict by anger, hostility, and self-assertiveness. If the outward expression, and hence release of these feelings, is inhibited by certain circumstances such as societal values which limit self-expression, the sympathetic nervous system, which is normally activated by anger, may remain chronically activated as a vent for expression of frustration. The sympathetic-like symptoms of anxiety and stress result, such as palpitations of the heart, increased perspiration, muscular tension, constricted pupils, and decreased activity of the digestive organs. Specifically, diabetes can result from chronically increased mobilization of carbohydrates, arthritis from increased muscle tension around joints and cardiovascular disease, hypertension (high blood pressure) and migraine headaches from increased blood vessel constriction. Thyroid hyperfunctioning may occur as a result of overstimulation of the thyroid gland or higher brain centers (pituitary or hypothalamus) which control the thyroid gland.

Similarly, a person may respond passively by running away (withdrawal). Again, if overt withdrawal is inhibited by societal standards or specific events, the parasympathetic nervous system may remain chronically stimulated as a symbolic expression of passive withdrawal. This results in overactivation of digestion and bronchial tube constriction, which manifest as ulcerative colitis, peptic ulcer disease, or asthma. For example, the typical ulcerative colitis patient reacts to stress not by action but by withdrawal. If this withdrawal is inhibited, the parasympathetic nervous system is activated. Increased gastro-intestinal activity produces diarrhea. In psychoanalytic theory this diarrhea represents a regression or withdrawal to times of infancy when the mother gave praise for having bowel movements.

Psychosomatic Medicine and the Central Nervous System. Another interesting example of mind-body interconnection which is included in the study of psychosomatic medicine is the inhibition of the central nervous system (CNS). The CNS is responsible for voluntary action—that which keeps a person voluntarily in communication with the external world. Inhibition of normal CNS responses can lead to a disorder called conversion hysteria. This illness is characterized by paralysis, loss of speech or loss of coordination, yet no physiological or pathological reason can account for the symptoms. The symptoms of conversion hysteria are associated with the voluntary and sensory systems, both of which are necessary to communicate with the outer world. Psychologically the person withdraws into fantasy (also directly controlled by the CNS). Unlike the ANS type disorder, the CNS ailment has no observable physiological disturbances such as ulcer crater or joint swelling. As soon as the conflict is resolved, the symptoms disappear, leaving no damage.

Autonomic Nervous System

	SYMPATHETIC	PARASYMPATHETIC
ORIGINS	Middle Portion of Spinal Cord (all thoracic and top three lumbar segments)	Brainstem (or Cranial Nerves) and Upper Sacral Segments of Spinal Cord
PHYSICAL FUNCTIONS		
Blood Pressure	Increase	Decrease
Heart Rate	Speeded up	Slowed down
Bronchial and Lung Passages	Dilates	Constricts
Iris Accommodation	Far Vision	Near Vision
Digestion	Diminishes Enzyme Secretion	Stimulates Pancreatic Enzymes
Stomach	Contracts Sphincter	Inhibits Sphincter Contraction
Intestinal Activity	Decreases	Increases
Muscles and Associative Blood Vessels	Constricts Arteries	Dilates Arteries
PSYCHOLOGICAL DISEASE	High Blood Pressure Migraine Heart Disease Thyroid Conditions Diabetes Melitus Arthritis	Low Blood Pressure Ulcer Ulcerative Colitis Asthma

Freudian Psychoanalysis. The Freudian psychoanalytic therapists especially penetrate into anger and repressed feelings associated with youth, so that the person can learn to identify these unconscious suppressions. Patterns of interaction with parents are discussed and sexual inhibitions and frustrations identified. In the psychoanalytic framework, a person passes through specific stages of development (called the oral, anal, phallic, latent, adolescent and adult periods). If conflict or inhibitions have occurred in any of these stages, certain predictable emotional patterns will arise. For example, if a young infant was not allowed enough time for sucking, or if, as some doctors now believe, the newborn was not breast fed, certain types of neurosis can develop. The baby might suck his thumb for an inordinate amount of time, the adolescent might bite his nails, the adult might overeat when under stress, or a businessman might develop a gastric ulcer in response to work pressures. In a similar vein, a toddler forced to toilet train before being emotionally mature enough may later develop severe constipation or diarrhea, anal compulsiveness, or peculiar obsessions like frequent hand washing.

In Freudian psychiatry, *libido* is the energy that drives and motivates a person. According to psychoanalysis, the main form of libido is sexual energy, and it is believed that unfulfilled libidinal (sexual) desires lead to unconscious conflict. Repressed sexual feelings and desires are considered by Freudians to be a major source of emotional problems, and interpretations of conflict tend to be oriented around this issue. For example, in Freudian theory if a woman dreams of a snake, it generally symbolizes that she is afraid of sex, since the snake represents a phallic symbol for the penis. When libido or energy is blocked because of sexual inhibitions, the mind and body become enervated. By liberating this sexual energy, the psyche and soma gradually become stronger and more balanced. By verbal expression of fears, thoughts, and dreams the repressed libido is released and can then be refocused into more balanced attitudes and thought patterns.

Inherent in psychoanalysis is the theory that human life consists of a struggle to counteract childhood or conflictual impulses and to uncover suppressed emotions and experiences. This system's major focus is on delineating the symptoms and signs of disorder. The real meaning of psychological health is not clearly established. Psychoanalysis describes positive health through inference by stating that "normal" people are able to maintain an intricate balance and identity (ego) between inner urges (id), which are often sexually oriented, and outer parental, environmental, or social demands (superego). The ego in this scheme is constantly being pulled by the id and the superego. A person who is able to keep both these influences from greatly disturbing daily functions is considered to be in relatively good psychological health.

Jungian Analytical Psychology. The Jungian approach to psychotherapy, called analytic psychology, is also used to treat psychosomatic illnesses. Analytical psychology tends to be more positively oriented in that it recognizes man's inner potential and need for a creative outlet. It also describes the deeper aspects of the mind, the unconscious, as reflected in dreams and universal symbols, and the close association between religious questions and psychology.

Dreams, symbols, and myths are "observable" reflections of the deeper levels of the mind, representing the mind's attempt to handle stress and emotional conflicts. Dreams often revolve around the day's unfinished business or represent attempts to express the repressed fears of daily living. They also, through their symbolism, give glimpses of higher states of consciousness. Dreams are thus manifestations of those hidden dimensions of life that normally evade our conscious scrutiny.

Jungian psychology recognizes the great power of the energy associated with the unconscious mind. If misdirected, this energy forms into certain patterns called complexes. Deeply rooted in the mind are specific images, fantasies, and myths that are common to all mankind. These "archetypes" in a sense reflect primordial patterns of psychic energy that give all people an interrelatedness by virtue of this dynamic force.

There are many similarities between this system and Freudian psychoanalysis which is not surprising since Jung was originally a student and colleague of Freud. There are also important differences, especially with regard to interpretation of psychological conflicts and events. Besides the relevance of problem identification and resolution, Jungian psychotherapeutics maintains that inner mental unrest represents the person's attempt to integrate various unknown qualities of his being. In this sense, emotional conflicts can be viewed positively as reflections of deeper aspects of a person's mind. Releasing and understanding these hidden mental forces can lead to great creative insight and experiences. For example, the snake in the previously mentioned dream might be interpreted as representing primal energy and the potential power for spiritual enfoldment, rather than simply the penis. The Jungian analyst would point out that the myths and symbols of the most ancient cultures and of philosophical systems like yoga commonly identify the symbol of the snake with the force that uplifts man to a more evolved state of awareness.

The Jungian therapist helps the patient understand that his problems, dreams, images, and emotions are all there to teach him, and that people throughout history have experienced the same joys, fears, and tribulations in their journey through life. This approach has many therapeutic benefits in that it helps the patient to identify with other people and to feel less alienated, and it provides a model that exemplifies the universality of mankind. This common reservoir of experiences is called *the collective unconscious*. It also enables the patient to view his conflicts as untapped inner resources which are there to teach him the lessons of life. By learning these lessons, he can continue to evolve and expand his consciousness.

Gestalt Therapy. Gestalt therapy can also be used in the treatment of psychosomatic ailments. In this approach, the person learns to experience directly the diverse aspects of his personality. Through experiencing and analyzing the component parts of a situation, the totality and inner meaning of the situation are perceived on a deeper level. The person actively participates in his own life drama by assuming various roles that reflect his inner mental state. For example, in the above-mentioned snake dream, the person would act out the roles of the woman who fears the snake, the snake itself, or perhaps the rocks the snake slides over or the clouds overhead, watching the whole scene. By assuming the emotions of each character, bits and pieces of underlying or unconscious attitudes, desires, and fears emerge. These are experienced directly and provide the patient with firsthand knowledge of his real feelings. The therapist guides, pushes, and prods the patient to go through and feel the Gestalt of each experience.

The Third Force

Abraham Maslow believed that human beings are continuously evolving, imbued with an inner impulse to "self actualize," and that they can reach "full humanness." What inhibits this expansion is a "defense against growth," as man fears not only his lowest attributes but also his highest potentiality. He evades his innate abilities and talents and circumscribes his mission in life and his destiny. In moments of "peak experience" he attains an ecstasy, perhaps expressed as a sense of merging with nature. Yet when the rapture subsides, an ambivalent and conflicting state sets in. He focuses on his negative side, passiveness, hostility, and greed. On the one hand, he loves and admires the world's great leaders, saints, and geniuses, as he loves those aspects inherent in himself. Yet he also feels in awe, uneasy, and inferior because the successful people also remind him of his imperfections. Hostility is the predictable and understandable consequence directed at those he admires, as well as at himself. He then sets up defenses to hide this anger or represses these feelings. The result is an evasion of both his negative qualities and his positive attributes.

Maslow also maintained that self-growth or mastery was predicated on adequate food, sex, sleep, and self-preservation. When these necessary life-sustaining requirements are adequately met, emotional energy is not dissipated but can be rechanneled for self-actualization or higher potentials. He would agree with the yoga concept that emotional problems stem from unfulfilled desires of these four basic needs.

While Maslow focused on concepts and theory of self-actualization, Roberto Assagioli's system, called Psychosynthesis, uses the yogic methods of meditation and concentration with the aim of enhancing transpersonal and spiritual development. Both systems focus on developing beyond the usual range of human capacities.

Psychotherapy and Meditation

The process of psychotherapy acts as a vehicle for unconscious mental phenomena to be brought into conscious awareness. Man stagnates and cannot grow if he remains ignorant of thoughts and emotions that create internal conflict. Hidden desires, memories, and fears can be analyzed and new understanding of inner dynamics can lead to the resolution of these problems. Verbal expression of anxieties often allows for release of tension. Interpreting dreams and fantasies can lead to an understanding of tendencies rooted deeply in the unconscious mind.

Change of attitude and habit can occur only if a person first understands the sources of his conflicts. Patterns of emotional reaction can be altered only if these patterns are first recognized. Free association and dream analysis are techniques that allow a person to objectively perceive and analyze the mind's contents and to identify enervating and distracting thoughts. Growth and expansion of awareness take place as the patient learns to integrate more of the unknown into the conscious, objective mind.

Psychotherapy, however, depends more on verbalization, which may distort the real meaning of the inner world, which is nonverbal in essence. The therapist's interpretation also leaves room for misconceptions and miscommunication because of his fallibilities. On the other hand, the meditative techniques of ancient medical systems work in a somewhat similar way, but meditation occurs on a nonverbal level and thus helps the practitioner to become independent of the need for an outside therapist.

Meditation also differs from most schools of psychotherapy because it leads the person beyond problem solving and conflict resolution. In certain meditation practices, while one observes the mind flow, he allows repressions to surface, and aspects of his inner being which were previously unknown to him become apparent. These memories, images, and thoughts are considered to be aspects of the unconscious mind because he was unaware or not conscious of their existence. This is similar to the growth process characteristic of psychotherapy when the patient learns how various unconscious conflicts and defenses lead to personality and emotional imbalances. When repressed and suppressed feelings and latent tendencies surface, they can be observed, analyzed, and released, leaving the inner psychic world clear. The distractions and inhibitions of random thought and fantasy are eliminated. The meditator considers them, not the end, but as preparation for a stage when the mind becomes an open, receptive field preparing to receive true inner knowledge and to experience the deepest, most subtle levels of existence.

The psychotherapeutic benefits of meditation can be more clearly understood by the following analogy. Man's mind is like the ocean, the surface representing the conscious mind with its innumerable fluctuating waves of thought and emotion. Lying beneath is the great ocean expanse analagous to the unconscious. The turbulence of the surface thought waves obscures the depths of knowledge underneath. The process of meditation calms the tumultuous ebb and flow of the sea's outer layer of wave activity. Bubbles and currents, which represent unconscious repressions and habits, are allowed to rise to the surface to be observed. Since no energy is supplied to suppress them, the bubbles gently burst and dissipate. This averts the creation under the surface of further increased pressure that can produce tidal waves (emotional storms). The ocean becomes quiet and still, and the deeper mysterious layer of the ocean floor (unconscious) can be observed and experienced. The individual wave (separate ego) is again merged with the greater ocean (universal Self). Tranquility and true knowledge result, and the individual experiences peace and bliss.

Clinical Applications

Holistic practitioners are in a unique position to observe how psychological conflict can lead to physical problems. Having a theoretical framework that is very broad based and includes several models of psychosomatic integration enables the clinician to evaluate emotional components of illness. The holistic physician also has diagnostic and therapeutic tools that include such diverse aspects as orthodox laboratory evaluation, written psychological testing, homeopathic case taking, and more traditional elemental classification found in Ayurveda, Chinese medicine, and yoga.

To effectively treat psychological problems, especially in association with physical ailments, physicians must individualize their therapy. For example, a blatantly schizophrenic or suicidal patient might need hospitalization or psychotropic medication. A person with phobias might need to undergo psychotherapy, learn biofeedback, and use homeopathic remedies. Someone with anxiety that seems to stem from eating specific foods might need a carefully planned diet and vitamin and mineral supplementation and an aerobic exercise program. An executive in a highly stressful work might need to learn relaxation techniques, meditation, and alternative methods of expressing frustration.

The holistic practitioner using psychotherapy needs to decide what approach to use. Jungian analysis might be used for a client who dreams in symbols and metaphors or has a spiritual outlook on life. A person whose conflicts seem to stem from early childhood might benefit from a psychoanalytic approach. A patient who can fantasize and role act might be helped by a Gestalt approach. A phobic person might be advised to use behavioral therapy. Nutrition, vitamin supplementation, exercise, relaxation, biofeedback or meditation, along with medicinal therapy including herbs, homeopathic remedies, or even drugs, could also be utilized concurrently with these psychotherapeutic techniques.

The therapy a holistic doctor decides to prescribe or undertake depends somewhat on his background, training, and expertise. A person trained in formal medicine might not have the necessary skills to personally conduct psychotherapy and might choose to refer a patient to a holistic psychiatrist or psychologist. On the other hand, a psychiatrist may decide to have a holistic internist thoroughly evaluate medical problems before beginning therapy.

A curious thing happens, however, as physicians practice holism and view things from a multidimensional perspective. The specialty distinctions begin to blur, psychological and medical techniques begin to blend, the psychiatrist enjoys doing more medicine and the family practitioner practices more psychotherapy. The clinician begins to understand what a rare privilege it is to be allowed to participate in and help treat patients from varying perspectives: how that person exercises, eats, dreams, thinks, acts, and feels. As a practitioner learns more about holism and applies that to human problems, he finds his responsibility grows as patients entrust them with ever more subtle aspects of their lives.

Conclusion

As psychology evolves in the humanistic direction, it seems that a real understanding of man's mind implies the recognition of the pivotal importance of his spiritual nature. This concept forms the very core of ancient medical and philosophical systems. It is no wonder that these philosophies have inspired men like Jung, Assagioli, and

Maslow to raise modern psychology to a level where it can begin to administer to all aspects of man's suffering: physical, emotional, and spiritual. The newer forms of psychology such as psychosomatic medicine and humanistic psychology have helped to popularize the principle of the unity of mind, body, and spirit in Western scientific medicine. In addition, humanistic psychology introduces the principle of growth as central to the pursuit of health. The philosophies of ancient medical systems such as yoga and Ayurveda shed light on the darkness and can help the psychologist address the questions: What controls the mind? What are the underlying causes of emotion? How does man's individual consciousness fit into universal consciousness?

10

Homeopathic and Medicinal Therapy

Definition and History

Homeopathy is a system for prescribing medicinal substances according to the "law of similars." This law dictates that the appropriate medicine for a sick individual is a substance which would create his exact set of symptoms if administered to a healthy person. The word *homeopathy* is derived from the Greek root *homeo* and means "like treatment of disease." The roots of the law of similars are ancient, having been described in the treatises of Hippocrates in Greece and by the Ayurvedic physicians in ancient India. Paracelsus, a fifteenth century physician, refers to the principle underlying the law of similars in his discussion of the Doctrine of Signatures. He stated, "You bring together the same anatomy of the herbs and the same anatomy of the illness into one order. This simile gives you understanding of the way in which you shall heal."[1]

---

[1]Coulter, *Divided Legacy: A History of the Schism in Medical Thought*, p. 432.

Homeopathy has been practiced throughout the world for the last 180 years since its rediscovery by the German physician, Samuel Hahnemann (1755-1843) in the early 1800s. Today homeopathy is widely employed in India, Mexico, South America, Germany, France, Great Britain, Russia, and other European countries. Homeopathy was introduced in the United States in 1825, and the American Institute of Homeopathy, the first national medical association, was founded in 1844. In the late 1800s, many homeopathic hospitals and medical schools existed in this country.

Law of Similars

Samuel Hahnemann, a practicing physician, became disillusioned by the dangers of existing therapies, such as the use of toxic doses of mercury for many ailments and the practices of blood letting and blood leeching. He turned to studying the pharmacology and healing principles of ancient and indigenous medical systems. In his studies, Hahnemann became interested in the curative effect that quinine had in the treatment of malaria. He experimented with quinine by ingesting small amounts over a period of time and eventually developed many of the symptoms of malaria. His conclusion was that quinine could cure malaria because it could create the typical symptoms of this particular disease. Thus, the law of similars was rediscovered by Hahnemann.

In light of this discovery, Hahnemann began a systematic study of many commonly known medicinal substances. He administered very small amounts of these substances to himself and other healthy volunteers over an extended period of time and carefully noted the symptoms that developed. This process of verifying the medicinal properties of these various substances is called "proving the medicine" and is derived from the German word *pruefung* meaning *test*. Through this work, a vast amount of knowledge was collected regarding the symptoms which these medicinal substances could produce in healthy people. According to the law of similars, one of these medicines could thus be administered and result in a curative effect in a sick person with an identical set of symptoms.

Health and Disease from a Homeopathic Perspective

A penetrating and thoughtful understanding of the concepts of health and disease is fundamental to comprehending the impact of the law of similars in medicinal therapy. The concept of health versus disease is not easy to define in terms of absolutes and may best be understood by examining the dynamics of the interaction of the individual and the environment. The nervous system, endocrine system, immune system, and other as yet undefined mechanisms catalyze the organism's response to environmental influences. Environmental pressures may variably include such factors as inherited genetic weaknesses, emotional stresses, mental or physical strain, injuries, environmental pollutants, bacteria or viruses, or nutritional deficiencies. If the individual's adaptive powers are strong enough to withstand the disruptive effect of these environmental stimuli, a state of health prevails. On the other hand, a disease state results if environmental factors stress the individual's adaptive powers beyond his limit to cope. Whether successful or not in the attempt to adapt, the organism is always striving for health. Consequently, in the effort to re-establish health, the symptoms of the sick person represent his attempt to overcome malevolent external stimuli. The symptoms are not the result of these stimuli but rather an expression of his reaction to the stimuli.

Although the homeopath may speculate as to what factors may be partly responsible in the origin of a disease, such as heredity, stress, bacteria, pollutants, or emotional elements, he acknowledges the existence of unknown factors which influence an individual's response to his environment and preclude a precise understanding of all that is responsible for the genesis of the illness. Though people vary tremendously in their ability to adapt to stress in the environment, the homeopathic prescriber is concerned with all of the apparent subjective factors which are associated with the onset of a person's health problems. Characteristics such as oversensitiveness, insecurity, lack of self-confidence, or laziness are important to know in the beginning in order to understand the nature of a person's illness and to choose the correct remedy. Illnesses are often seen to date back to precipitating events which resulted in grief, worry, disappointed love, or childhood neglect.

Homeopathic philosophy contends that, from the onset of life until death, the individual is reacting with his environment in the most intelligent way possible. The homeopath, like the Chinese and Ayurvedic doctor, believes in the existence of a vital healing force which is always moving in the direction of greater overall balance for the whole person and which is clearly articulated in every mental, emotional, and physical symptom. The symptoms of an illness are a clear expression of this intelligence at work, attempting to re-establish a state of health.

The homeopath indirectly obtains information about the cause of disease by studying the body's reaction to it. This reaction is depicted by the symptoms such as fever, cough, diarrhea, or pain. The healing response to disease, as depicted by the symptoms, is ultimately the most crucial information in terms of choosing a remedy that is similar to these symptoms. Based on the law of similars, a medicinal substance is chosen which reinforces the symptoms that are representative of the mind-body attempting to heal itself.

Not only can homeopathic remedies treat disease, but they can also prevent it. Even if no specific diagnosis of the group of symptoms exists and all diagnostic studies are within the normal range, treatment can be instituted. This is because the way the symptom complex manifests is an accurate expression of the forces of the disease process. There are signals or sensations in general, or in specific body areas, long before actual tissue damage takes place. By administering the appropriate homeopathic remedy, a disease process may be halted before it progresses to pathological changes. In this respect, homeopathy can be a preventive medical system. For example, Western allopathic doctors generally disregard the liver as being the source of illness unless liver enzymes are elevated. Only when these blood-test changes occur, or when pathological destruction is proven by X-ray, ultrasonic scan, or biopsy, will medicine be given. Even then, few drugs are considered effective in such diseases as hepatitis or cirrhosis. The homeopath, on the other hand, recognizes that certain changes in mind and body herald underlying liver dysfunction. Even if the liver enzymes are normal, symptoms such as a heavily coated tongue, vague abdominal pain in the right upper side, sluggishness in the morning, and a melancholy mood or hypochondriasis all suggest liver malfunction. The homeopathic physician prescribes a remedy based upon the totality of these symptoms so that the liver functioning can return to normal. In this way, symptoms are eliminated and potential diseases are prevented. Similarly, other vague or poorly treated illnesses, such as viral infections or allergies, respond well to homeopathy, using the symptoms which the mind-body produces as a guide to prescribing.

It is fundamental in homeopathy to view the symptoms of an illness as a curative response by the entire organism. This means that, despite the presence of symptoms in various part of the body such as the skin, lungs or joints, there is nevertheless only one illness present. Each symptom is related to another, forming a single psychophysiological condition. In homeopathic treatment, the one medicine which can produce the entire constellation of symptoms in a healthy person is administered to cure the ailing person.

Law of Proving

The law of proving is the systematic verification of the law of similars. As earlier described, healthy people take a remedy over a certain time period and report their subjective symptoms and sensations. When the same symptoms are found to be common to a specified proportion of experimenters, they are considered the "proving" of that remedy. Hahnemann stated, "There is . . . no other possible way in which the peculiar effects of medicines or the health of individuals can be accurately ascertained—there is no sure, no more natural way of accomplishing this object, than to administer the . . . medicine experimentally, in moderate doses, to healthy persons, in order to ascertain which changes, symptoms, and signs of their influence each individually produces on the health of the body and of the mind."[2]

Approximately 1,500 different remedies have been proven over the years. Plants, minerals, and extracts from animals, such as snake venom, are among the many agents used in the preparation of homeopathic remedies.

Proving a remedy involves the observation of the unique mental, emotional, and physical symptoms peculiar to each medicinal substance. Food cravings and aversions, mood fluctuations, memory and concentration, sleep quality, and sensitivity to external stimuli such as weather—all are carefully recorded, along with the areas of bodily discomfort and any factors which either increase or decrease the discomfort. In the proving of a remedy, mental and emotional symptoms are often reflected in physical signs and symptoms. For example, the remedy *Sulphur* is associated with a personality that tends to be easily vexed, argues about philosophical matters, and is quite irritable and disorganized. Physical symptoms correspond with those of the mental sphere; hence the patient's emotional volatility manifests in a red, flushed, "hot" appearance, profuse sweat, and skin eruptions. He is often haggard, disheveled, and dirty, qualities which correspond to his mental disorganization.

The specific mind and body symptomatology that each

---

[2]S. Hahnemann, *The Organon of Medicine*. New Delhi: Jain Publishers, 1974, p. 189.

medicine is capable of producing during the proving has been collected and compiled in books called *Materia Medica*. These books are complemented by other books called repertories which are compendiums of symptoms, listing the substances that cause each physical and psychological symptom.

This detailed knowledge of the symptomatology of medicinal substances provides the ways and means for a high degree of specificity in prescribing for each individual. The importance of sharp selectivity in prescribing medicinal substances has been emphasized by the Nobel Prize winning microbiologist René Dubois: "It is obvious that the sharper the selectivity of a biologically active substance, the greater the probability that it will be innocuous for cells and functions other than the one for which it has been designed. In other words, a substance is more likely to be therapeutically useful if it acts almost uniquely against a structure or an activity peculiar to the organism or function to be affected."[3]

Two children who suffer with middle ear infection (otitis media) might provide an example of specificity in homeopathic prescribing. One child may appear extremely irritable and oversensitive and may be sweaty, thirsty, and susceptible to drafts, wishing to be well covered with blankets. His ear pain may be worse with cold applications and better from warmth. Homeopathically prepared *Hepar Sulphuris Calcareum* (calcium sulphide) produces these symptoms in a healthy person and would act curatively in this particular case. The other child may display a mild and weepy disposition, wanting to be held and comforted. Lack of perspiration, thirstlessness, and wanting to be uncovered and outside in the open air may be apparent. The ear pain may improve with cold packs and become worse from the application of heat. *Pulsatilla* (windflower) would be needed to cure this child and *Hepar* would probably not

---

[3]R. Dubois, *Drugs in Our Society*, Baltimore: John Hopkins, 1964, pp. 38-39.

help at all. The reaction of the vitality as expressed through perspiration pattern, thirst, and reaction to weather and temperature are totally opposite in these two children. The selection of the remedy which is most similar to the symptoms will lead to a rapid and lasting cure of the illness.

Law of Potentization

When Hahnemann first began treating people according to the law of similars, many of the medicines he used were potentially toxic substances such as mercury and arsenic. To prevent toxic reaction to these substances, they were sequentially diluted before being administered. Though toxicity was reduced by dilution, there was also a concomitant decrease in therapeutic effect. As a result of his extensive knowledge of ancient and indigenous medicinal systems, Hahnemann was aware of a method of increasing the activity of a medicinal solution by vigorously shaking it in its container, so he methodically shook his medicines after each dilution. He found that, as the toxic properties were steadily reduced with each dilution, the therapeutic efficacy increased with the shaking—a seemingly paradoxical effect. It is this method of increasing therapeutic effect with each sequential dilution by shaking which is known as *potentization*. The potency of small amounts of medicinal substances is not novel, as is demonstrated in the case of thyroid hormone; free thyroid hormone in the human is one part per 10,000 million parts of blood plasma. Potentization also provides a means for releasing medicinal qualities from supposedly inert substances such as common table salt.

In the actual preparation of the potentized medicine, one part of the medicine is either diluted with nine parts of alcohol and water solution or ground with nine parts of milk sugar (lactose). This mixture undergoes vigorous shaking (succussion) or grinding (trituration) to produce what is called a 1x potency. One part of this mixture is added to another nine parts of alcohol and water solution or lactose, and the shaking or grinding is repeated, resulting in a 2x potency. Potencies may range from 3x to 500,000x. If the dilutions are one part remedy to one hundred parts of either alcohol and water or lactose, then this is called a "c" (centessimal) rather than an "x" (decimal) potency.

Potentization is controversial because, according to the laws of chemistry, by the time the 24x potency is reached, there are few if any molecules of the substance left in the solution. However, potencies such as 200x or 1000x act more quickly, are effective over a longer period of time, and thus require fewer doses than the 3x or 6x preparations. Homeopaths do not exactly know how these potencies work. They speculate that the process of potentization liberates the energetic essence of the substance and that the solvent (alcohol and water solution or lactose) acts as a template or vehicle in which the energy of the medicine is imprinted and preserved. This concept of a template can be better understood in light of the effects that pressure has on ice crystallization of freezing water. The late Harvard Physics Department Chairman, P. W. Bridgman, reported different crystallization patterns for water freezing at higher altitudes than for water freezing at lower altitudes. When the ice from the higher altitude was melted and refrozen at lower altitudes, the crystallization pattern of the higher altitude was maintained.[4] The effect of pressure on crystallization was demonstrable and indelible. Perhaps the homeopathic remedy exerts a similar effect on its solute.

Critics of homeopathy suggest that homeopathic medicines could only exert a placebo effect because the high dilutions do not contain measurable amounts of the medicinal substance. However, the proving of a homeopathic medicine using dilutions greater than 24x are a strong argument against this. It is unlikely that many *different* people would

---

[4]P. W. Bridgman, *The Physics of High Pressure* (Magnolia, MA: Peter Smith, n.d.)

experience the *same* set of symptoms from a given medicine if the medicine were simply a placebo.[5]

Vital Force

The concept of the vital force is fascinating and integral to understanding homeopathic medicine. This concept helps to explain the dynamics of how the potentized remedy interacts with the sick person to effect a cure. Vital force is not a biochemical entity. Rather, it is the energetic essence that complements man's physical form. This energetic essence or vital healing force represents the difference between a living and a dead person. It is that quality which animates living organisms and constantly seeks homeostasis in an inherently intelligent way.

All aspects of nature, whether mineral, vegetable, or animal, have an underlying energy pattern. Homeopathic remedies are derived from these three kingdoms. The energy pattern or vital force of these remedies is seemingly enhanced by potentization.

Homeopathy maintains that the vital force permeates all levels of man's existence, body, mind, and spirit, and is analogous to the prana of yoga or the chi of Oriental philosophy. Man is viewed as a dynamic whole with the vital force acting as the integrating factor. Healthy people have a particular quality or pattern to their vital force, but when they become sick this subtle essence is distorted. Still, even during illness this healing force reacts in the most self-preserving manner, and its plan is clearly articulated through the symptom complex.

In homeopathy, energy qualities of the remedy, as revealed by the proving of the remedy, are matched with the

[5]D. Ullman, "Principles of Homeopathy." *Co-evolution Quarterly,* Spring, 1981, p. 66.

unhealthy person's energy qualities, which are manifested by physical, mental, and emotional symptoms. Through the law of similars, a cure is effected. Perhaps the similar vibratory qualities of the remedy and the sick person produce a harmonic resonance which helps to balance the patient's vital force.[6]

Western medical science describes the defense mechanisms of the human organism as a physiochemical phenomenon. Antibodies, lymphocytes, gamma globulin, and interferon are thought to somehow interact to protect and rid the body of internal or external disease agents. The factors that underlie their functioning, however, remain elusive. Homeopathic theory states that it is the vital force which underlies these defense mechanisms. If the vital force is aligned, then the defenses maintain homeostasis; if the life force is disturbed, illness results.

Orthodox medicine acknowledges that disease can result from the defective functioning of "physiologic energy," which generates heat, enhances metabolism, and along with various enzymes is responsible for maintaining important physiochemical reactions in the body. These latter energy reactions are responsible for the transmission of nerve impulses and production of ATP or cellular energy from oxygen and glucose. However, Western medicine does not recognize that disease and disharmony can manifest on a more subtle energy level. As a consequence, no treatment is directed towards eliminating illness that reflects energy imbalances.

The energy referred to in homeopathy is more fundamental and subtle and underlies the physiologic energy of the body. Without this deep energy, the biochemical reactions could not occur. There have been isolated verifications of this subtle energy such as Kirlian photography and acupuncture experimentation, which have objectified electromagnet energy fields around living things. However,

---

[6]G. Vithoulkis, *The Science of Homeopathy*, p. 96.

technology has not been developed to a sufficient degree to analyze this vital energy. We cannot assume from that, however, that the energy is not real. Two hundred years ago people would have scoffed at the idea of electrical energy, and fifty years ago the concept of nuclear energy might have seemed preposterous. As technology advanced, these energies were isolated, channeled, and reproduced with amazing rapidity and skill. Eastern medical traditions and a few branches of Western medicine have discovered that the underlying subtle energy is not only real, but is also fundamental to health and disease. In time it may be recognized in traditional Western medicine.

Hering's Law of Cure

Constantine Hering (1800-1880) is considered the father of American homeopathy and was responsible for many valuable contributions to medicine. Based upon his observation of mental, emotional, and physical symptoms as a barometer of the overall health of a person, he was able to measure improvement or deterioration of health. Hering's "Law of Cure" states that:

(1) Healing moves from the deepest and most vital parts of the person (mental and emotional states; vital organs) to the most superficial and least vital parts of the person (joints; extremities; skin).
(2) Healing moves from the upper parts of the body to the lower parts.
(3) As healing progresses, symptoms disappear in the reverse order of their appearance.

Healing moves from the most vital to least vital parts of the person. The natural direction of cure is always outward or centrifugal as the organism attempts to establish homeostasis by externalizing disease. Although a person may complain of one or several limiting physical complaints when first coming to the doctor, careful scrutiny often reveals mental or emotional problems that actually preceded the physical problem. It is rather uncommon to see a person with a physical problem without a pre-existing or concomitant psycho-emotional component such as anxiety, depression, or irritability. That mental and emotional symptoms frequently precede the appearance of physical symptoms was also observed by practitioners of other systems, such a Ayurveda, yoga, and Chinese medicine, and this is the contention of modern psychosomatic medicine, as we have seen.

The physical symptoms can be seen as a means for decompressing pressures that build up internally and limit mental and emotional freedom. Seen from this perspective, the physical limitation is the result of the healing force's ability to externalize the disease process and preserve the integrity of the more vital and inner mental and emotional life. Mental and emotional health may be considered more crucial than physical health. An extreme example is a person who is paraplegic as a result of multiple sclerosis but is relatively balanced in mental and emotional functions, who may be healthier and able to enjoy a higher quality of life than a schizophrenic with few physical limitations but with a delusional and paranoid mind.

There is also a hierarchy in the body in terms of which organs are more or less inner and vital. A clear example is seen in the phenomenon of shock, either due to hemorrhage of blood or massive infection. To sustain life in shock, blood is shunted away from the less important organs to the most vital ones. The outer skin becomes cold and blue due to the redistribution of blood, and the intestinal tract and kidneys shut down. The preponderance of blood flow is to the brain and heart, the two most vital organs that are necessary to sustain human physical life.

The homeopathic remedy is prescribed with a thorough understanding of all mental, emotional, and physical symptoms. Through its effect on the vital healing force, the remedy acts as a "channel" for smooth, efficient transmission of the disease process from the mind to the body and finally out of the organism. If the first sign of an illness appears in the mental and emotional realm, treatment must take these symptoms into account. The person must first feel better subjectively if cure is proceeding in the proper direction. Physical symptoms, such as a skin rash, may get worse as the cure is taking place and the disease is being externalized to the least vital parts of the organism.

If medicinal treatments are given for ailments without a thorough and integrated understanding of their origin and without an understanding of the whole person and the predictable patterns of disease progression or regression, the natural defense mechanism may be suppressed and a poorer state of health may result.

A typical problem often seen by homeopathic doctors is infantile eczema. Allopathic doctors usually treat these skin eruptions with cortisone creams, but the underlying process and individual symptom pattern is neglected. Topical treatment of eczema is often suppressive in nature and forces the problem inward. If the suppression is chronic, the skin symptoms may improve while the destructive force shifts to the internal organs. Classically, the lungs are affected and bronchial infections and possibly asthma result. In fact, homeopaths believe that in most cases asthma and eczema are the same disease. The eruptions and skin appearance so characteristic of eczema can be pushed further inward, affecting the mental state of the child, resulting in symptoms such as irritability and temper tantrums. The centrifugal healing response is suppressed and a centripetal progression of disease supervenes. The deeper organs, and finally the mind, are affected because there is no way to release the disease through less harmful areas, such as the skin. The original process becomes more deeply entrenched (as the eczema is suppressed and the disease has spread from less vital areas to more vital ones). In the process of cure, the homeopath would carefully observe the progression of symptoms. True cure would be said to occur only if the mental state first improved and then the asthma abated.

The external skin symptoms may reappear and would improve later in the course of treatment as the centrifugal healing response is re-established.

A disease process can be viewed as an obstacle which is encountered, similar to a wall that a hiker must climb to continue his journey. As he attempts to climb the wall, a boost may be given and the obstacle easily overcome, just as the homeopathic remedy assists the vital force's attempt to overcome obstacles to health.

On the other hand, a person can be pushed to the bottom as he attempts to climb over the wall. The force is applied in a direction opposite to the desired movement. This matching of vector forces in opposite directions is similar to the dynamics of allopathic drug actions. Although it may temporarily reduce the discomfort of the climb, being pushed to the bottom of the wall does not help the hiker continue his journey since he is simply avoiding the problem. Similarly, the allopathic drug will not help the defense mechanism overcome challenges. That wall may have to be met sooner or later. If one is pushed to the bottom repeatedly, weakness and frustration may ensue and the wall may become insurmountable. When this analogy is applied to health, it is seen that after repeated suppressions the defense mechanism becomes progressively weaker, the symptoms of illness are continuously present, and a chronic disease state exists.

Cure moves from above downwards. Homeopathic physicians carefully observe the progression of disease, either in "provings" or after the administration of remedies. Since symptoms move from higher areas of the body to lower areas during the the curative process, eczema that is being treated with a homeopathic remedy, for example, will often descend from the eyelids to the elbows to the knees before disappearing. Subjective sensations such as pain or tingling also progress in a downward direction when the patient is improving. The reverse direction will often be found in cases where eczema or pain worsen.

Symptoms disappear in the reverse order of their appearance. Detailed analysis of symptom regression has shown that as the patient improves, the symptoms that appeared last are the first to disappear, while those symptoms which appeared earlier, disappear later.

The reverse of this law is also true in that disease progresses from superficial and less vital body parts to deeper and more vital areas; and that disease spreads from the lower parts of the body to the uppermost parts. These laws exemplify that the nature of disease is not random or mysterious. Natural laws govern all forms of life, and it is illogical to assume that man's health is an exception.

Chinese medicine also recognizes that disease progresses in certain patterns, similar to the homeopathic law of cure. The Chinese system asserts that disease moves from yang (lower and external parts of the body) to yin (upper, inner parts of the body). Cure of illness occurs in the opposite direction: yin to yang. When illness moves towards the yang, a person is said to be regaining health, but when disease turns yin or inwards, the patient is regressing. This is exactly equivalent to the homeopathic theory, though the two systems were founded in completely different ages in entirely different parts of the world. Homeopathy and Chinese medicine also concur that cure moves in the reverse order from the original appearance of symptoms. A quote from the *Yellow Emperor's Book of Internal Medicine* exemplifies that point.

On the first day the injury of the cold is received by the great Yang. Therefore the head and the neck are in pain; the waist and back become rigid. On the second day the region of the "sunlight" receives the disease. The "sunlight" controls the flesh, its pulse supports the nose and is connected with the eyes. Thus when the body is hot (feverish), the eyes ache, the nose is dry and the patient finds it impossible to rest. On the third day the region of the lesser Yang receives the disease. The region of the lesser Yang controls the gall bladder. Its pulse follows the flanks and is connected with the ears. Thus the ribs and the chest are in pain and the ears turn deaf. Now the three regions of Yang and the arteries have received the disease; however, it has not yet entered the viscera and therefore one can produce perspiration and terminate it.

This description continues until, on the sixth day, all parts of the body are affected by the disease. If at that time both the blood and the vital substances cease to move about, death follows. If, however, the patient remains alive after the crisis on the sixth day, there will be gradual improvement, during which the organs recover in the same order in which they were affected, so that, on the twelfth day, all symptoms of the disease disappear.[7]

Allopathy

Allopathy is the form of medicinal treatment which is used by most doctors in this country. It is a system for prescribing medicinal substances according to principles other than the law of similars. Allopathy is derived from the Greek root *allo* and means "other treatment of disease." Hahnemann coined the word to describe the treatment based on the law of contraries and all other treatments not prescribed strictly in accord with the principles of homeopathy.

The forerunners of today's allopathic doctors were certain physicians of Greek and then Roman eras. They gradually replaced the importance of the abstract and undefinable vital healing force of the organism with a reciprocal emphasis upon understanding the individual in terms of physiochemical laws. They began to view the body as a material and mechanical entity and sought to understand it through the laws of physiology, chemistry, and physics. The

---

[7]Huang, *The Yellow Emperor's Classic of Internal Medicine*, p. 51.

role of the vital healing force was neglected because it could not be measured with these mechanistic tools.

Galen was a second-century physician whose extensive work and writings did much to establish allopathic theory as we know it today. Galen postulated a concept of disease based upon his knowledge of the body obtained through anatomy and physiology. He postulated that the vital healing force existed only as it was expressed in the various organs of the body, with each organ having its own behavior and manifesting certain qualities which could be rationally studied. This approach obscured the functioning of the organism as a whole and instead focused on the many parts. Galen's teachings, with emphasis on the organ systems of the body as the key to understanding and treating disease, is easily recognized in modern allopathic medicine. Modern medicine is a highly subdivided profession with its various kidney, heart, or lung specialists who study disease processes as they eventually appear in these organs, and who use the physical laws of the scientific method.[8]

Health and Disease from an Allopathic Perspective

Allopathic medicine has traditionally tried to understand the cause of disease by examining its effects. Bacteria, tumors, and toxic metabolites which are found in diseased tissues are implicated as causes of disease, whereas they might actually be the result of disease when viewed from the homeopathic perspective. Experimental science, using the same laws of chemistry and physiology as allopathic medicine, supports the allopathic approach as truly "scientific." However, the subtle factors which influence the appearance of disease, such as the individual's lack of internal resistance

---

[8]Richard Grossinger, *Planet Medicine*, (Boulder, CO: Shambhala, 1982), Chapter 10.

to environmental stresses, are disregarded in this methodology. In other words, factors which are important in the
cause of disease but which cannot be studied by rational and
reductionistic methods are overlooked by allopathic medicine. Also, since allopathy is oriented toward diagnosis using pathology as a guide, diagnosis and treatment of many
states of ill health are vague or non-existent when tissue
studies and laboratory tests are normal.

The body's innate intelligence, expressed through the
symptoms that it produces, is ignored as instead the body's
physiochemical properties are analyzed. The symptoms are
not viewed as a reaction to disease but as the result of disease. They are considered aberrant by the allopath and, in
accord with the law of contraries, medicinal substances
which have an opposite effect are administered to eliminate
the symptoms. However, medicines applied according to
this principle go "against the grain of the wood" from the
homeopathic view, in that they oppose or suppress the
organism's own healing response. Repeated exposure to
these treatment principles, or even their occasional application in an individual with weak powers of resistance, may
lead to further weakening of the individual's defense
mechanism. It is clear that (1) a fever is a response of the
defense mechanism against infection; (2) a cough is a means
of eliminating mucus and irritants from the lungs; (3) tears
remove irritants from the eyes; (4) increased intestinal activity in food poisoning resulting in diarrhea or vomiting is a
means of removing toxic substances. These physical symptoms (fever, cough, tearing, diarrhea) and, in fact, all physical symptoms clearly communicate the person's adaptive
reaction to a disease process. Suppression of these symptoms
may eventually lead to more severe limitation of health and
chronic disease.

Psychiatry is one branch of traditional allopathic medicine which has some appreciation of the problems that may
result from suppressing symptoms. Psychotherapists con-
tend that thoughts, feelings, and emotions that arise from
the conscious and subconscious mind represent the person's

reaction to psychological trauma. Greater mental and emotional health ensues as these thoughts and feelings are recognized, accepted, and integrated with greater understanding into the person's life. On the other hand, denial of strong feelings leads to the development of defenses which may suppress these feelings into deeper layers of the conscious and unconscious mind and eventually lead to more severe mental and psychological limitation. Physical symptoms should not be interpreted differently from psychological symptoms. However, the allopathic model has reduced the view of the individual from a vitally integrated whole into a mechanistic group of parts. Many different illnesses can exist in the same individual, with a "skin doctor" managing one and a "heart doctor" another. Emotional problems are relegated to psychiatrists, as the result of a poor understanding of the interrelatedness of physical and psychological health.

Allopathy's real strengths are in the same areas where this system has focused its emphasis. Anatomy, physiology, biochemistry, and pathology are highly developed. Technical aspects of surgery and laboratory diagnosis are highly sophisticated. The weakness of the system is its poor understanding of the dynamic and energetic nature of the human organism in disease progression and regression. Ultimately, the result has been the adoption of a fragmented system of medicinal therapeutics.

In traditional medical training in this country the approach to therapy is generally considered to be medicine first (i.e. allopathic medicine) and surgery second. This means that since medicine is relatively less invasive than surgery, medicine should always be the first choice to control a health problem if it is effective. In our practices we have amended this rule to homeopathy first, allopathic medicine second, and surgery third. The reason for this is that homeopathy actually strengthens the sick person, which is preferable to drugs which do not enhance the person's resistance to disease but merely strive to reduce or eliminate the most distressing symptoms.

Obviously, surgery remains the first choice for illnesses such as some injuries from accidents, gunshot wounds, and other such forms of trauma. It can also be helpful as an adjunct to managing chronic disease, for example replacement of scarred heart valves resulting from rheumatic fever, total hip replacements in advanced arthritis, or removal of a cancerous tumor. But, although the surgery may be successful, it may be naive to consider the person "cured" without carefully assessing his life style, eating habits, and ways of coping with stress, which may have lowered the person's resistance and allowed the cancer, arthritis, or heart disease to begin.

Allopathic medicines can be helpful in the nonsurgical management of disease. Some examples include the drugs used to resuscitate people in cardiac arrest, medicines used to treat advanced pathologic diseases such as insulin in diabetes and digitalis in heart failure, and antimicrobial drugs such as penicillin used in bacterial meningitis or other life-threatening infections.

The physician should *selectively* make use of *all* therapy that is available and appropriate. The first choice of the holistic practitioner should be modalities that strengthen the patient, resulting in less susceptibility and more resistance to disease. These are the therapies which are discussed in this book. Therapies which are not vitalistic in their approach such as surgery and allopathic medicines, should be a second choice except if specifically indicated in life-threatening situations, or in medical conditions which are extremely advanced, or in diseases in which vitalistic therapy proves ineffective.

Clinical Applications

We have seen that both Eastern and Western cultures have developed schemes or patterns for understanding and describing man in terms of his emotional, physical, and mental characteristics. In the East, this organization of characteristics is a direct reflection of the origin and the order of the universe, or macrocosm. Man is seen to originate from within the universe, and as a microcosm of the universe he is subject to its laws of interaction and transformation.

Chinese and Ayurvedic medicine and yoga philosophy all depict man and everything in the universe as made up of various combinations of basic elements, as already discussed. For the Chinese these are metal, earth, water, wood, and fire, which interact in a balanced or unbalanced way to produce harmony or chaos, health or disease. The Tridosha of Ayurvedic medicine consists of vat (air and ether), pit (air and fire), and kaph (earth and water), while yoga philosophy divides prana into the tattvas: akasha, vayu, tejas, apas, and prithivi. In all these systems the body and mind of man are seen as being composed of and nourished by various elements. Many correspondences can be found among these different systems, even though each developed separately.

In the Western world in medieval times the humors of blood, phlegm, choler, and melancholy, and their associated temperaments of sanguine, phlegmatic, choleric, and melancholic expressed a similar attempt to understand and categorize the fundamental essences that form and influence man. This scheme, too, has correspondences with the other ancient systems. The hot-tempered and fiery choleric temperament is easily recognized in the fire element of Eastern cultures. Likewise, the indolent, calm, and self-possessed phlegmatic temperament is comparable to the Eastern water element. Other similar parallels can be drawn, though these are the most striking.

The technological advances of the Western world have allowed man to examine himself in minute detail. The use of the microscope and the field of embryology have enabled man to study himself from the time of conception. A researcher named W. H. Sheldon has found some support for a theory of human types. Embryology divides early human life, before recognizable form has appeared, into three major tissue types: ectoderm, endoderm, and mesoderm. The ectoderm gives rise to the skin and nervous system, the endoderm to the digestive linings, and the mesoderm to the skeleton, muscles, and organs of the body. People of slender build and nervous temperament might be considered to have a predominance of ectomorphic tissue control and are termed *ectomorphs*. These types are similar to the vat, or air, elemental types in their characteristics. We might think of obese and lethargic people as having their metabolic energy poorly focused in the endodermic or digestive tissue and there they might tend to be overly, though unevenly, nourished. These types are termed *endomorphs* and are very similar to the kaph or water types. Finally, the well-built and muscular mesomorphic type, somewhere between the previously mentioned types in terms of body structure, might be thought of as having predominant mesoderm or muscular tissue focus. The mesomorph resembles the pit or fire elemental type in mental and physical characteristics.

In homeotherapeutics the triad of remedies *Sulphur, Calcarea Carbonica*, and *Lycopodium* is frequently used. These complement each other and are effective in treating a very wide range of physical, mental, and emotional problems. In *A Dictionary of Practical Materia Medica*, Dr. John H. Clarke wrote, "It is absolutely essential to a correct appreciation of the Homeopathic Materia Medica that these three medicines *(Sulphur, Calcarea* and *Lycopodium)* should be thoroughly known, as they are in a sense the standards around which the rest are grouped."[9]

The fiery and irritable *Sulphur* patient with warm, sweaty hands and feet clearly exemplifies the fire element of Chinese and Ayurvedic systems, as well as the Western choleric and mesomorphic types. The unevenly nourished, cold, dull and flabby *Calcarea Carbonica* patient is the same as the earth and/or water elements and the

---

[9]John A. Clark, *A Dictionary of Practical Materia Medica*. New Delhi: Jain Publishing, 1978, p.329.

phlegmatic or endomorphic element. Finally, the depressed, thin and withered, gassy *Lycopodium* patient closely resembles the air, ectomorphic, and possibly melancholic type. The following chart is a comparison of the different systems of categorization of human characteristics based on physical, emotional, and/or mental patterns.

Chart of Type Similarities

Chinese Elemental Types	Yoga Tattvas	Ayurvedic Tridosha	Homeopathic Remedies	Western Physiognomy	Medieval Humors
Air	Akasha	Vat	Lycopodium	Ectomorph	Melancholic
Wood	Vayu				
Fire	Tejas	Pit	Sulphur	Mesomorph	Choleric or Sanguenaric
Water	Apas				
Earth	Prithivi	Kaph	Calcarea Carbonica	Endomorph	Phlegmatic

This attempt to understand man within the context of the world of which he is a part underlines his inseparability from nature and from the laws of cause and effect. Though from different systems, the similarities of these observations are striking considering the diversity of their time and place of origin. These basic types help to point out the simplicity amid the seeming complexity of nature, while at the same time showing the subtle differences between people. Recognition and acceptance of this uniqueness of human expression is the first step in appreciating the importance of addressing this uniqueness in the origin and treatment of disease. The individual is a dynamic factor in the disease equation rather than an inanimate victim.

For example, an obese, apathetic person, always chilly, who repeatedly develops sore throats in cold and damp weather could likely need a homeopathic remedy like

Calcarea Carb, a treatment to strengthen the kaph or water element. A thin, red-faced person intolerant of warm weather who has recurring sore throats might better be treated with *Sulphur* homeopathically, and would benefit from treatment intended to regulate the pit or fire element in her constitution. To use the same treatment (for example, penicillin) for both of these people because of the common symptoms of the sore throat, may be shortsighted; the two people are quite different in most other respects. These differences are the fingerprints which help identify the underlying susceptibility to disease. This example highlights the difference between the modern allopathic and more traditional healing systems in terms of diagnosis and treatment. In allopathy the treatment is indicated as soon as the priniple focus is discerned, and individual uniqueness, which characterizes the person's susceptibility to the disease, is ignored. The treatment may kill bacteria or reduce the inflammatory response but do nothing to directly strengthen the patient. In traditional schools of medicine, definitive treatment depends on understanding and correcting the underlying weakness within the person because this has led to the acute problem.

Conclusion

Homeopathy is truly an example of holism, with a single remedy being prescribed for a person based on a thorough understanding of all aspects of his mental, emotional, and physical health. The homeopathic patient must carefully observe symptoms, noting factors or circumstances which aggravate or ameliorate his ailments. His feelings and general mood are important because each remedy is associated with particular emotional characteristics. He must observe his reactions to stimuli, both with respect to his total being and specifically with respect to his individual parts. This process helps the individual to experience previously unknown aspects of his inner nature as he learns to observe his own biorhythms, cravings, aversions, and habits. Recurring dreams, specific fears, and peculiar idiosyncrasies become apparent. Thoughts and emotions that create pain or discomfort in certain organ systems become obvious. Homeopathy, like meditation and psychotherapy, helps the individual to learn about himself. The knowledge gained through this self-observation aids an individual in the process of bringing into conscious awareness elements of his existence that before were happening on an unconscious level. In homeopathy the patient's observation of symptoms is equally as important as the action of the prescribed remedy.

If man is viewed as a microcosm, a reflection of nature and the universe, then all elements that comprise this macrocosm are also found within man's body, mind, and spirit. Both the physician and patient begin to see the world in the form of patterns because each remedy provides a different, complete picture of life. Each picture is like another piece in the universal puzzle. As the puzzle gets filled in, life becomes less mysterious and frightening. It becomes apparent that the remedy is a symbolic, though practical, representation of the unconscious mind. Homeopathic knowledge and treatment combined with other holistic systems can lead an individual to experience this great unity. Life then becomes more controllable, more comprehensible, and more exciting.

IV

Union of Ancient and Modern Systems of Holistic Medicine

11

Yoga: A Complete Holistic Medical Model

Yoga as a system is a highly developed empirical science. Its benefits, physical, emotional, and mental, have been repeatedly verified through thousands of years of systematic experimentation with specific techniques and observances. Inner yogic knowledge was passed on from teacher to student long before man discovered the means for mass communication. This informal mode of transmission has led to many variations on the common theme of inner exploration of psyche and soma. Cultural imperatives, geographical barriers, and societal idiosyncrasies have caused people both to develop theories and to interpret their inner observations in different ways. As a result, experiences of the higher realms of consciousness vary, allowing for varying approaches to meditation and differing techniques in such areas as chakra development. Yet, a few common principles underlie all the great systems of the world—whether from the religious traditions of the Judaeo-Christian, Moslem, Buddhist, Hindu, or Taoist, from the indigenous cultures of the American Indian or African tribesman, or from highly developed philosophical systems like yoga, Vedanta, or Existentialism. These principles may be stated in dissimilar words and different metaphors may be used to describe them, but underneath is the common esoteric knowledge that mind and body are one, that man and the universe are interrelated, and that the struggle for life with all its pain and joy represents a journey of self-discovery.

Because of its completeness, depth, and practicality, yoga represents perhaps the most eminent of all holistic and preventive health care models. Yoga concepts embody a practical framework around which a holistic health approach can be organized. These include: (1) the five sheaths of consciousness and (2) the chakras.

The Five Sheaths of Consciousness

According to yoga, the progression of disease can be understood in the context of the *koshas* or the five sheaths. Disease begins in the deepest and most subtle level of unconsciousness. All physical ills or emotional disorders and mental disease have their origins in this deepest level of consciousness. As man disassociates from his true nature, where the innermost Self is one and the same as the universal Self, misdirected desires to possess the objects of the world begin to emerge, and disorder moves outwards. Disease then progresses to less subtle parts of the unconscious mind, the conscious mind, the energy sheath, and finally to the body.

The five levels of consciousness are conceptualized as existing from gross external levels to more subtle internal ones, the outer being more dense and obscuring the finer, less material inner layers. Associated with each level is a specific type of awareness. These five levels of consciousness are called sheaths because of their concentric arrangement, although they all interpenetrate one another. The philosophy of koshas or sheaths represents a model of preventive and holistic health which offers both conceptual theory and pragmatic treatment approaches into which various other therapeutic systems of healing can be integrated.

The five major sheaths of consciousness that may be treated are the body or physical sheath, the energy or pranic sheath, the mind, the intellectual or unconscious sheath, and the blissful or transcendental sheath. Within the last sheath lies the Self, which is the source of all the other levels. When disease occurs, treatment can be directed towards any of these levels.

These sheaths form a continuum, and all levels are interdependent. Because man exists simultaneously on all these levels, the cause, diagnosis, and treatment of disease must be ascertained with respect to the five sheaths. In order to truly be considered healthy, a person should be balanced in accordance with all these multitudinal expressions of consciousness. Yoga science teaches many practical techniques and health practices to help bring harmony to each level of existence.

All the systems and therapies presented in this book can be integrated into the yogic sheath concept. A particular therapy may be employed to effect a cure at different levels within an individual. Nutrition, for example, works primarily on the first sheath, the physical body. Yet, it must be remembered that because the models presented in this book are holistic, any therapeutic modality will also affect the other levels of consciousness. Therefore, nutritional therapy, for example, will also affect the mind. If a person doesn't choose good quality of food or is deficient in certain minerals or vitamins, his nervous tissue and brain will not function optimally. This can cause imbalances in nervous system transmission or hormonal levels, which in turn affect behavior and emotional expression.

Following is a synopsis of the five sheaths, from the grossest to the subtlest, with a description of what therapies can be incorporated into each level.

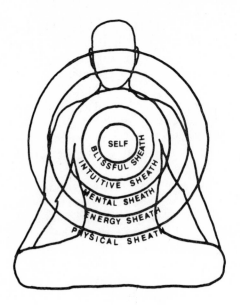

Physical Sheath

The first level, the *physical sheath*, includes the physio-anatomical structure of man. Called the *Annamaya kosha*, it is the focus of some of the aspects of the holistic therapies of nutrition and physiotherapy. In addition to specific yoga-related disciplines, other areas of health care which may be associated with this sheath are nutrition, exercise, physio-therapy, allopathic drug therapy, surgery, and some ayurvedic and herbal medicines.

Changing to a vegetarian diet is a natural tendency when a person begins to practice the science of yoga. Foods that are naturally grown and lack chemicals and artificial ingredients bring about a sense of well-being and result in less internal toxicity. Diets which do not include meat help facilitate a sense of physical lightness and mental clarity. Diseases related to high fat intake are minimized, including hypertension, heart disease, and stroke. Other ailments, such as certain cancers and arthritis, are statistically less common in vegetarians.

Hatha yoga, which occupies the third step in the Raja Yoga system, helps bring about greater body awareness, relaxation, flexibility, balance, strength, and concentration. As a person works with hatha yoga, he becomes aware of bodily tension and where it is held. Yogic cleansing techniques help to cleanse the body of excess waste from the eyes, skin, upper respiratory mucus membranes, lungs, stomach, liver, colon, kidneys, and bladder. The body becomes less congested and the excretory functions work properly. Cell metabolism operates more smoothly since there are less waste and excretory by-products to interfere with normal tissue physiology. Diseases such as colds, allergies, colitis, cystitis, and asthma, become less serious or are cured.

Breathing exercises have many beneficial effects on the physical level. Over a lifetime people develop bad habits and do not breathe with maximum efficiency. Shallow and irregular respiration, accompanied by toxic fumes in the air, exacerbates such diseases as asthma, pneumonia, and bronchitis. Breathing techniques can prevent disease and hasten the cure of these respiratory infections. Abnormal lung growths are caused by both environmental pollution and chronic degenerative habits such as faulty nutrition or smoking. Here again, breathing exercises may act preventively, stimulating stagnant pulmonary areas where abnormal growth predominates.

Breath cleansing techniques contribute to the relief of such common disorders as allergies, sinusitis, tonsillitis, and laryngitis. Deep, smooth breathing assures that a sufficient amount of oxygen is supplied to all the tissues, including brain, heart, and muscles, re-establishing homeostasis and physiological equilibrium.

Elementary breathing exercises such as diaphragmatic breathing lead to self-regulation by increased control of the autonomic nervous system and an expanded ability to direct the emotions. By cultivating the skill of breath awareness, "standing back" for a few moments and impartially viewing the nature, direction, and rhythm of the breath flow, a person can begin to transform his consciousness and personality. He will come to understand that certain emotional stimuli or thought patterns alter the inspiratory and expiratory cycle. He notices, for instance, that he holds his breath while under stress, for example in studying for exams, and consequently feels tired and weak. Or he may breathe rapidly with short bursts while driving in heavy traffic, becoming fidgety and nervous. Suppressed anger often activates the sympathetic nervous system which is associated with chest breathing, constriction of arteries, and hypertension. Diaphragmatic breathing, through its effect on the autonomic nervous system as well as on thoughts and emotions, helps to balance the psychological cause (anger) and the physiological expression (vasoconstriction) of this problem.

If a person has practiced and experienced the benefits of smooth, effortless breathing while performing pranayama techniques, he can adapt this fluidity to times of stress that are associated with breathing irregularity. Irrational feelings or scattered thinking are then brought under more conscious control. Slowly he learns to watch his respiratory cycle with such efficiency that the emotional extremes are minimized or prevented.

Energy Sheath

The second sheath, *Pranamaya kosha*, is the energy body. Stress management therapy and homeopathy are directed to work on imbalances on this level. Because disease manifests in the energy fields of man, treatment methods which are directly focused at this level of existence can effectively eliminate suffering. Areas of health care associated with this sheath are biofeedback, relaxation techniques, pranayama techniques, homeopathy and acupuncture.

Energy, whether called libido, psychic energy, the vital force, prana, or chi, is the link between the body and the mind. It is the life force that animates the human organism. The major transmitter of energy from the external world is the breath and, to a lesser degree, food. We have seen that homeopathic remedy balances and brings about order to this vital force. Since energy is the link between the mind and body, imbalances in the energy field often reflect mental disorder and predate body pathology. Before mental disease can produce physiologic changes, the disharmony must first pass through this intermediary energy level. Conversely, suppressed physical illness will also show manifestations in energy patterns before affecting the mind or emotions. Homeopathic medicines act directly on the vital energy level because, through the processes of dilution and attenuation (potentization), they have been refined to match the level of vital energy functioning.

Chinese acupuncture therapy, as discussed earlier, also works on the energy level. Needles or finger pressure are applied on pathways that transmit energy flow. These meridians have no real correlation with nerve pathways but are similar to the yogic idea of nadis. By stimulating certain points, a balancing of energy flow is facilitated in distant organs. Pain reduction or anesthesia is also possible through acupuncture therapy.

On an energy level, the uneven breath results in an erratic flow of prana. Physiologically, irregular breathing influences every cell of the body by its effect on oxygenation and blood flow and on the central nervous system, the autonomic nervous system, and the emotions. With conscious control of the breath, a person can learn to observe and direct the amount and quality of energy entering the body. Through slow, deliberate practice of simple breathing techniques such as diaphragmatic breathing, a person learns to discern which irregularities of the breath flow reflect particular illnesses, how certain states of mind adversely affect breathing patterns, and also how to redirect and guide the breath to create harmony between the mind and body.

Yoga psychology states with physics that energy (prana in yoga) exists in one of two forms—manifest or potential. Yoga sees an endless interchange between the two: involution, the process whereby potential energy transforms into manifest matter, and evolution, representing the reverse process. Potential energy functions at a higher and faster vibrational level than manifested form. Higher states of consciousness can be understood within this concept as representing different stages of this latent or potential force. Pranayama helps the aspirant to cleanse the inner currents of obstructions and to increase his capacity to tolerate and channel the great amount of energy associated with the highest stages of consciousness.

Specific yoga pranayama or breathing techniques in association with stress reduction techniques and relaxation exercises help to facilitate smooth and efficient transmission of pranic energy, between the outer and inner worlds as well as within the subtler bodies of the practitioner of yoga.

It seems reasonable that part of the control afforded by breathing exercises and yoga in general may be due to the pacification of the sympathetic system. This control is accomplished through correct upright posture, which removes tension from the two sympathetic cords along the spinal canal. It is also facilitated through activation of the opposing parasympathetic system by diaphragmatic breathing and control of the nerve plexuses associated with the chakras. For example, special control of the solar plexus, which is mainly supplied by the right vagus nerve, seems essential to achieve parasympathetic control. The conscious relaxation which results from diaphragmatic breathing also effects the pacification of the large sympathetic glands, the adrenals, which are located in the area of the solar plexus.

Parasympathetic nerves (found in the nose, pharynx, stretch receptors of the lungs, and chemoreceptors of the carotid body) are stimulated by pranayama techniques. Parasympathetic nerve plexuses are also found in the major centers in the body that correspond with the chakras, which will be discussed presently. In fact, many yogis who are versed in anatomy and physiology state that it is control and stimulation of the parasympathetic system, primarily through the right vagus nerve, that is essential and actively promoted through pranayama. Activation of this system through breathing exercises and deep concentration is generally associated with relaxation and slowing down of physiological processes.

After mastering the parasympathetic nervous system, the practitioner who advances in breathing exercises may gain greater control of the hypothalamus, where the parasympathetic nervous system finally sends its nerve impulses. From the central controlling station of the hypothalamus, control of the connecting limbic system (emotions), cerebral cortex (thoughts and intellectual ideas), pituitary gland (endocrine gland activities), rhinencephalon (instinct), appetite center, and body temperature center may be gained. This may explain how pranayama may lead the advanced practitioner of yoga to control of his body, mind, and senses.

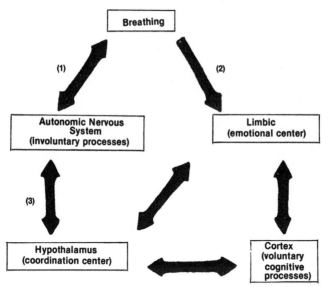

How Breathing Affects Voluntary, Involuntary
and Emotional Processes

---

(1) through vagus-parasympathetic nerves (nose receptors, lung stretch receptors, cardiac-celiac plexus, carotid sinuses)

(2) nose (olefactory nerve to rhinencephalon)

(3) parasympathetic nerve

It is important not to confuse these physiological mechanisms with those of the more subtle pranic energy pathways. They are separate, parallel systems, operating simultaneously, yet at different vibratory levels. Prana underlies all physical functioning, for yoga philosophy states that without prana there would be no physiology or life. By controlling the parasympathetic system, sympathetic nervous system, spinal and cerebral centers, the physical body is calmed and, in a sense, purified, allowing the more subtle, underlying parallel pranic forces to be observed, directed, and regulated. By controlling these various nerve systems, unconscious aspects of a person's being come into conscious awareness. As control of pranic forces occurs, expanded states of consciousness are experienced.

Physics is beginning to confirm what modern psychology and ancient systems purport, that matter is simply condensed and slowly vibrating patterns of energy which can be discerned by man. Seen from this perspective, the entire universe is really different forms of energy at different states of manifestations and levels of vibration. This underlying dynamic energy is the integrating link between the physical, mental, and spiritual realms of creation.

Since mankind's physical and mental being is a microcosm, a reflection of nature's macrocosm, all vibrations and forces within the human organism also exist in the outer world. The universe is, in a sense, an ocean of prana and each person a small pranic wave in this vast sea—individual, yet part of the whole. By identifying, controlling, and thoroughly knowing his own pranic essence, he understands the subtle forms of all other waves; the entire ocean is comprehended. His individual ego merges with all other egos and he becomes permanently identified with the whole. He becomes a truly universal being.

Mental Sheath

The third sheath is the mental body (*Manomaya kosha*), the vehicle of conscious control. Most Western psychotherapy deals with this level of ego re-integration, as do certain yogic concentration techniques. More specifically, the models of psychosomatic medicine and the meditational therapies of yoga and Chinese philosophies can be incorporated in the mind sheath. Areas of health care associated with this sheath are most schools of Western psychotherapy and yogic concentration techniques which emphasize nonattached observation of the thought flow. The most important purposes of the techniques associated here are to help strengthen ego in the Freudian sense of conscious decision-making.

From the deeper levels of consciousness one can both observe and control the more exterior levels. Most people have awareness of their physical body. As sensitivity increases, a person learns to sense energy flows within the body and, by careful observation and analysis, can learn to locate energy blocks which underlie physical muscular tension. Sensitive individuals can even predict oncoming physical ailments by experiencing alterations in energy flow or through changes in the breath, the main vehicle for energy transmission. An even deeper function is the mind. The way a person thinks often determines the way he uses his body. By mentally sending messages to his body and observing energy flow, a person can consciously learn to relax muscular stress and help cure such tension-related diseases as high blood pressure and migraines.

Intuitive Sheath

The fourth sheath, the intuitive level (*Vijnanamaya kosha*) encompasses all the holistic therapies that the more superficial mental sheath does. It relates to certain unconscious levels of the mind and to altered or expanded states of consciousness in which one feels unified with all. Here a refining of the intuitive nonverbal faculties is found, allowing deeper unexplored levels of the human psyche to be integrated within the individual.

Areas of health care associated with this sheath are the

techniques of free associations of Freudian psychoanalysis, dream analysis of Jungian psychology, active and passive imagination, and all schools of deeper meditation.

Certain forms of meditation can help a person to observe the character of his mental and emotional life. Through witnessing the flow of thoughts and feelings, he may then acknowledge that the persistent fears or obsessions with which he identifies may prevent him from feeling potential inner strength. When the mind is quiet and fears or obsessions diminish, this strength can be contacted, rendering him less vulnerable to previously challenging circumstances. This strength facilitates a feeling of completeness that allows the person to adapt to changes in the environment without feeling threatened. The completeness leads to a feeling of wholeness within and less dependency on the ever-changing environment for nurturance.

Meditation, when applied to actual living situations, can enable a person to feel the full range of emotions but also maintain a sense of impartiality and neutrality. When a stressful event occurs, his reactions can be viewed with an inner objectivity, and his emotions can be directed in more constructive ways. Thus he experiences emotions more acutely yet does not become enslaved by them.

The process of meditation sets the stage for self-awareness and expansion as the meditator directs his focus of concentration inwards. As he sits silently, he withdraws from sensory perceptions, he learns to objectively view the thoughts, fantasies, and images of the mind. By witnessing the internal mental world with neutrality or detachment, he becomes aware of disturbing thought patterns and how they lead to emotional and physical suffering. This problem identification is similar to that found in psychotherapy and is the first step in catalyzing change in habits and attitude.

After witnessing these troublesome thought and emotional patterns, the practitioner of meditation realizes the fleeting, ever-changing character of the mental field. Acknowledging the impermanence of thought makes him aware that there is an element of unreality associated with the patterns of the mind. He comes to know a quiet, calm, and centered part of himself that lies beyond the mind. He then can observe the mind and use the mind as a tool, yet not become identified with it. The meditator learns to "let go" of transient desires and vacillating emotions. He becomes less attached to meaningless mental events, freeing mental energy for more creative purposes and expanding awareness.

Blissful Sheath

The fifth level, the blissful sheath *(Anandamaya kosha)*, is characterized by perfect equanimity—after the power of discrimination has led a person to a state of truth, knowledge, and bliss. Within this last sheath is the soul or Self. When an individual has established himself and totally identifies with this level, he has attained enlightenment (samadhi). Only through the consistent practice of meditation over a long period of time is this state reached.[1]

Only holistic practices that teach advanced meditational techniques apply to this fifth sheath. Yoga meditation based upon chakra concentration and raising of the primal energy *(kundalini)* are among the most comprehensive and sophisticated of all meditation teachings. The goal is to create a state of peace, harmony, deep understanding, love, and pure joy.

When the conscious mind has been cleared, the mind can concentrate on a single point, such as a mantra. This is a sound repeated mentally, although repetitions or chanting aloud also help to concentrate the mind. As the meditator advances, his concentration becomes absorbed with the sound. Co-ordinating this sound with the breath flow helps the body, breath, and mind function as an integrated whole. The mantra's vibration is a subtle manifestation of the deepest levels of inner existence. Thus, by constantly remembering the mantra vibration, a person is led inwards

---

[1]Rama, Ballentine, and Ajaya, *Yoga and Psychotherapy: The Evolution of Consciousness*, Introduction.

Kosha Associations

KOSHA	TREATMENT/THERAPY[1] (OR PREVENTIVE APPROACH)	DISEASE	RAJA YOGA LIMB	ASSOCIATED CHAKRA

Physical Body (Anamaya)	Nutrition
	Vitamins/minerals
	Exercise
	  Passive
	  Hatha Yoga
	  T'ai Chi
	  Manipulation
	  Massage
	  Physical Therapy
	  Aerobic
	Herbs
	Drugs[2]
	Surgery
		Pathology of Systems:
		musculo-skeletal
		organ
		blood/lymph
			Yama (restraints)
			Niyama (observances)
			Hatha (postures)
				Anal (Self-preservation)
				Genital (Sexuality)

Energy - Breath (Pranamaya)	Homeopathy Acupuncture Pranamaya[3] (Breathing Exercises)	Functional diseases (symptoms without changes in physiochemistry) Psychomatic	Pranayama	Solar Plexus (Energy or power issues)
Mental - Conscious (Manomaya)	Biofeedback Counseling Psychotherapy (behavioral)	Anxiety Neurosis Phobia	Yama Niyama Pratyahara (Senses withdrawn)	Heart (Emotions consciously felt)

KOSHA	TREATMENT/THERAPY (OR PREVENTIVE APPROACH)	DISEASE	RAJA YOGA LIMB	ASSOCIATED CHAKRA
Intuitive - Unconscious	Psychotherapy Analytic Jungian Gestalt Dream Analysis Visualization Concentration Meditation	Personality disorder Schizophrenia	Dharana (Concentration)	Throat (Creativity and receptivity of unconscious thoughts and feelings)
Blissful - Superconscious (Anandamaya)	Concentration Meditation		Dhyana (Meditation)	Brow (Intuition and higher states of consciousness)
Self - Center of consciousness	Absorption in deepest meditation		Samadhi (Absorption)	Crown

1. This chart should not be interpreted in a rigid way. It is meant to function as a guide for understanding how the koshas are related to therapy, disease, and other forms of yoga philosophy.

2. Drugs can be used to treat mental diseases, but their primary focus of action is on the physical level since drugs work on the mind by altering the body's chemistry.

3. Breathing can also affect health of the body, but its initial effects are on the energy level. This idea applies to other treatments, such as nutrition's affect on the mind, homeopathy's effect on various levels of the mind, and biofeedback's affect in helping physical diseases.

towards the original seed of all existence. Finally, the whole meditative process culminates with the total elimination of mundane distractions and complete absorption with the true Self. The narrow confining "I" is cast off, and one merges with the Self to attain perfect peace, knowledge, love, and bliss. This state has many names—enlightenment, illumination, atonement, God or Christ consciousness, self-realization, samadhi, nirvana, the Tao—all of which reflect the same culminating experience.

The center of consciousness, also called the Self, soul, or God-realization, is contained within all the sheaths. This is the pure light of consciousness which is obscured by the many shades of the various sheaths. As the inner sheaths become slowly penetrated and mastered by long sustained meditation in combination with other holistically oriented health practices, the pure light can be experienced, leading to absolute truth, knowledge, and enlightenment.

The unconscious mind, characterized by mental images and intuitive understanding, often determines and underlies thought patterns and both mental and physical habits. As consciousness is directed inward towards the blissful and superconscious states, one realizes that these subtle domains are truly what lies behind life itself. It is from here that the ability to watch thoughts and actions stems, and this is where meditation leads as the process of watching and observing with passive awareness is strengthened. Piercing through the final sheath, the center of consciousness is realized, and one glimpses that all manifestation arises from this deep level.

The Chakras

The chakras provide an important yogic framework which helps illustrate the interconnections among the various levels of consciousness. Though based on the synthesis of Vedanta philosophy, the yoga philosophy of Patanjali, and the ancient Tantric system, the concept of chakras offers a theoretical construct useful in modern therapeutic systems.

There are many conceptions of the chakra system. In deep meditation individual practitioners experience the configuration of the chakras as an energy pattern. Different people from various traditions may perceive them in ways that differ in some subtle aspects. The system used here is borrowed from the meditational systems that developed around the philosophy of Vedanta and the Samaya school of Tantric yoga, the latter being a form of totally internal visualization and mantra repetition. Swami Rama's books *Yoga and Psychotherapy* and *Living with the Himalayan Masters* present an excellent and detailed overview of the chakras, koshas, and philosophical systems of yoga and Tantra.

Chakra means *wheel* in Sanskrit. As the wheel is characterized by movement of spokes emanating from a central hub, the chakras represent a focal area of energy (of a subtle kind not yet known to science) surrounding a central point from which motion and energy originate. These superphysical wheels represent force fields that transform energy from its source (consciousness) into various physical, mental, and spiritual qualities. Concentration and meditation on an energy center stimulate these qualities and also affect physiological functions associated with that center. For example, focused, sustained awareness on the heart or fourth chakra can improve lung and heart functioning and also strengthen the qualities of love and compassion.

The chakras are located in the junctures where the ida and pingala, the two major energy currents, crisscross over the sushumna, which lies within the central area of the spinal canal. Yoga maintains that the light of consciousness passes through the sushumna. This light is dynamic and vibrant, and as it moves, energy is transmitted through different of the centers. The nadis are the major conduits of energy transmission between chakras.

These seven centers represent intense fields of physiological, electromagnetic, mental, and spiritual energy. Yoga teaches that the body and mind are actually built along the lines, swirls, and eddies of this energy, which is transformed as it passes through these psycho-physical stations. The physical organs are activated by the subtle pulsations of this force at each center. The various functions and special forms of energy whirling through the seven centers of consciousness determine the physiology and psychological qualities characteristic of that chakra. A different level of consciousness is associated with each chakra, each higher center representing a more evolved state of activity and awareness.

Yoga teaches that the symbols associated with chakras are not just abstract representations. Just as iron filings form specific patterns reflecting the electromagnetic field of a nearby magnet, the energy that flows through the transforming stations (chakras) of the body also form particular configurations, reflecting the energy field of that chakra. Thus, the heart chakra, symbolized by the Star of David surrounded by twelve lotus petals, actually mirrors the energy formation peculiar to that area. As the formation blossoms, sending pulsations and vibrations outward, not only shapes but specific colors, tastes, qualities (earth, water, fire, air, space), and personality characteristics are manifested. As the energy form penetrates further into the gross physical world, the organs and body structure are formed.

Though not themselves physical, the seven chakras are positioned along the spinal column of the physical body. It is interesting to note how closely they correspond to the locations of the major nerve plexuses and endocrine glands, especially since the chakra concept evolved, through subtle means of self-observation and meditation, long before details of nervous and endocrine functions were known. Each center is associated with either an endocrine gland or nerve plexus. A deficient or misdirected focus of energy at a particular chakra will present ailments characteristic of the functions of that chakra. The lower centers generally represent the outer sheaths (body, vital energy, and conscious mind), while the higher chakras represent the more subtle, inner sheaths of higher awareness (unconscious, super-conscious, and Self).

The first chakra is located at the base of the spine and is related to the coccygeal plexus and large bowel. Yoga teachers maintain that it is associated with the psychological qualities of support, survival instincts, and self-preservation. If energy is balanced in the first chakra, a person will have a strong, solid framework on which to build his consciousness. Pathology here often manifests psychologically as paranoia or physically as bowel disorders such as constipation or ulcerative colitis.

The second chakra at the level of the genitals is associated with the sacral plexus and gonads, and issues of sexuality are prominent. Disturbances here often present as sexual identification problems, venereal disease, or sacral back pain.

The third chakra is opposite the navel, near the spine, and is related to the celiac plexus (solar plexus). Concerns

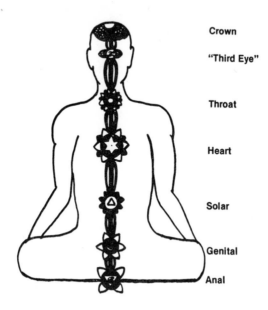

Crown

"Third Eye"

Throat

Heart

Solar

Genital

Anal

The Chakras

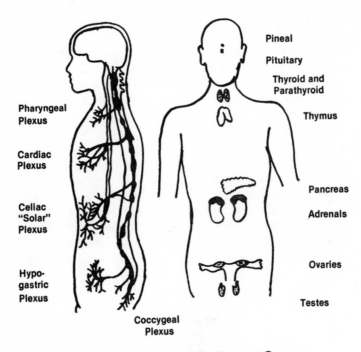

Pharyngeal
Plexus

Cardiac
Plexus

Celiac
"Solar"
Plexus

Hypo-
gastric
Plexus

Coccygeal
Plexus

Pineal

Pituitary

Thyroid and
Parathyroid

Thymus

Pancreas

Adrenals

Ovaries

Testes

Nerve Plexuses and Endocrine Organ Relationships to Chakras

at this level are said to deal with digestion and metabolism, as well as the emotional characteristics of dominance, submission, and assertiveness. Duodenal ulcers, diabetes, and other complaints of the abdominal viscera originate here. The common problems of compulsive eating and superiority or inferiority complexes can often be traced to misguided direction of energy at this point.

The fourth chakra is located at the level between the shoulder blades, near the heart, with the cardiac plexus of the autonomic nervous system being closely affiliated. Issues of love and empathic emotion are related to this center, and pathology might manifest as apathy, asthma, and cardiovascular disease.

The fifth chakra is across from the thyroid gland and

deals with communication, nurturing, creativity, and receptivity. Diseases such as hyperthyroidism, chronic tonsillitis, globus hystericus, and lack of creative expression are common imbalances.

The sixth chakra is found between the eyebrows. It corresponds to either the pineal or pituitary glands and is the seat of intuition and integration of awareness. Deeper mental disorders such as schizophrenia may be associated with inadequate integration at this center of consciousness.

The seventh and highest chakra, which is found at the vertex of the brain, may be associated with the pituitary or cerebral cortex, both of which coordinate physiopsychic functioning. When consciousness is centered here, the deepest sheaths and the Self are directly experienced.

The Yoga System as a Model for Treatment

The major principles of yoga can be consistently used in a general medical practice. It is a very practical method to analyze problems as occurring on physical, energy, emotional, mental, philosophical, or spiritual levels. The therapeutic approach which incorporates the sheaths and chakras will become clear if we examine how specific disorders or imbalances can be treated from this perspective.

The discussion of effective treatment on each level is not meant to be a complete survey of all possible therapies. The purpose is to illustrate a holistic approach in the framework of yoga for the treatment of various health problems. For example, a common complaint of patients is fatigue and lethargy. Using yoga as a model would enable the practitioner not only to study the problem systematically but also to see how the various levels of consciousness interact. For the physical perspective, appropriate blood tests and laboratory procedures would be ordered to rule out such factors as anemia, hypoglycemia, hypothyroidism, or tumor. A dietary evaluation might disclose a deficiency of a

Chakra Associations

CHAKRA	ORGAN	NERVE OR GLAND ASSOC.	PHYSICAL QUALITY	PHYSICAL SYMPTOM, DISEASE	PSYCHO-SPIR. QUALITY	PSYCHO-SPIR. SYMPT. OR DIS.	ELEMENT
Anal	Colon Anus	Coccygeal Plexus	Elimination	Ulcerative Colitis Constipation	Self-Preservation Support and uplift body and mind	Lethargy Paranoia	Earth
Genital	Genital Organs (Penis, Vagina)	Hypo-Gastric Plexus (Testes, Ovaries)	Reproduction Sexuality	Venereal Dis. Urinary Tract Infections	Procreation Sexuality	Sexual Preoccupation Sexual Identity	Water
Solar	Digestive Tract	Celiac (Solar) Plexus Adrenal Glands	Digestion Metabolism (Stress reaction)	Ulcers Diabetes Poor Digestion	Aggressiveness Submissiveness	Inferiority/ Superiority Complexes Energy Storage Center	Fire
Heart	Heart Lungs	Cardiac Plexus	Circulation Respiration	Heart Disease Asthma	Love	Apathy Hatred of Overemotionalism	Air
Throat	Thyroid Upper Respiratory (Ear, nose throat larynx)	Pharyngeal Plexus Thyroid	Speech and Communication Metabolism Growth Senses	Hyper-thyroidism Upper Resp. Infections	Communication Creativity Nurturance	Inhibition of Feelings Lack of Creativity	Ether
"Third Eye"	Pituitary or Pineal Gland Eyes	Pineal Gland	::::	::::	Intuition Higher States of Consciousness	Schizophrenia	:::
Crown	Brain Cerebral	::::	::::	::::	Samadhi God-Consciousness Self-Realization	::::	:::

specific nutrient such as Vitamin B or calcium, and foods high in these substances or a supplement would be prescribed. Energizing yoga postures could be taught, especially those that stimulate the solar plexus (or third chakra area) such as the cobra, spinal twist, or peacock. Vigorous breathing exercises such as Kapalabhati or the Complete Yoga Breath could be used to enhance vigor. (See Appendix.) Thus, the concept of the sheaths and chakras provides a practical therapeutic model for integrating a therapeutic approach to the whole person on all levels of consciousness. It demonstrates that treatment need not be directed only toward eliminating the physical aspects of disease and its negative, harmful qualities. Rather, treatment can be utilized to enhance the positive, growth-oriented aspects of human life.

How a person addresses his state of health or disease helps to determine the possibility for well-being. For example, he can adopt the attitude that it is possible to learn from all situations, whether positive or negative, and that both health and disease offer opportunities for increased understanding. On the other hand, he can view illness as a fearful, unpleasant, and burdensome condition. From a holistic perspective, if a person assesses the experiences of illness as positive or as a means of liberating blocked habits, thoughts, and emotions, then he has matured and evolved. Becoming receptive to those thoughts, emotions, and habits which accompany or precede disease is an essential primary step. After gaining such insights, a person can then prevent or alter potentially destructive attitudes which lead to conflict and disease.

We have chosen five diseases to discuss in the next chapters—asthma, hyperthyroidism, ulcers, lower bowel diseases, and skin disorders. All these are considered to be psychosomatic from the psychoanalytic perspective (as described in the sections on stress and psychotherapy). We have chosen these illnesses for a specific purpose. Our intent is to illustrate the direct correlations between mental and emotional conflict and problems with physical health. This does not mean that other diseases which are not classified as psychosomatic will not respond to a holistic approach. In fact, almost any ailment—even illnesses such as infections and back problems that are manifested primarily on a physical level with little or no mental and emotional involvement—can be treated holistically. In such instances, therapies which are directed primarily at the physical and/or energy levels would apply. The yoga concept of the sheaths is an integrating approach to therapy which is flexible and adaptable to each person's unique needs.

Using yoga philosophy as our model, we will analyze the five diseases from an integrated approach. Our attempt is to illustrate that a disease can be understood and treated both from the perspectives of the ancient holistic models (Chinese medicine, Ayurveda, and yoga) and from the modern holistic models (nutrition, movement, stress theory, psychotherapy, and homeopathy). It is also our intent to show that all these therapies have similar underlying principles and that they can be synergistically used in analyzing and treating an ailing person.

12

Asthma

Mr. D. is a thirty-one-year-old man who first developed asthma in 1971. His medical history included eczema as a child and nasal allergies in his late teens. He described himself as "a person who doesn't like getting out of control" and said he is passive, fearful of responsibility, and worries about being taken for granted. He had recurring feelings of guilt and was in general depressed, discontented, and withdrawn. He tended to withdraw from conflict and, while often feeling angry inside, had great difficulty in expressing this emotion. He had specific problems communicating with his parents and found it impossible to argue with his mother. In fact, anger coming from his mother would precipitate an asthmatic attack because he interpreted anger as rejection. He found that the fetal position helped relieve his shortness of breath.

This is a typical example of an asthma patient. In this chapter we will look at asthma from the various levels of consciousness, incorporating the yogic concepts of the sheaths and chakras and the various ancient and modern therapies presented in this book. We will end the chapter with a description of a treatment plan for this patient which incorporates all aspects of his disease.

Causes of Asthma

Physiologically, asthma is characterized by a constriction of the muscles that surround the bronchi, with resultant narrowing of the bronchial tubes. The friction produced by air passing through the narrowed passageways creates the characteristic asthmatic wheeze, which is usually worse on exhalation. Excess mucus accompanies the bronchial constriction because the tiny mucus-producing goblet cells become overactive due to irritation. There are biochemical substances mediating the bronchial constriction and excess mucus secretion: the parasympathetic hormone acetylcholine and, in allergic cases, histamine.

Psychosomatic medicine offers an interesting explanation of how emotional conflicts can lead to asthmatic conditions. According to this theory, the asthmatic individual is often excessively dependent upon his or her mother or another adult who assumes a maternal role, and unconsciously desires to "merge" or "reunite" with this person.

There are two major ways in which a person deals with uncomfortable emotional impositions such as an overbearing and demanding parent. One is to *actively* rebel and fight. If this rebelliousness is frustrated by a punitive parent, then there may be symbolic activation of the sympathetic nervous system, which stimulates *active* internal functions like raising blood pressure. The other mechanism for dealing with an overbearing parent is passively withdrawing and avoiding the influence. If this is prevented by the parent (or society) making more demands, symbolic activation of the parasympathetic nervous system can be triggered, which stimulates *passive* internal functions, including constriction of the muscles that surround the bronchi. This occurs in the case of asthma.

According to psychosomatic theory, the asthmatic's unconscious wish for reunion would confer protection and eternal love, and this is often symbolically expressed in recurring dreams of water (amniotic fluid). Some people feel very uncomfortable with these dependent feelings and fantasies, and consequently they create defenses. The asthmatic defense against maternal dependency is to avoid or run away in an attempt to escape these obsessional and confusing feelings. This withdrawal response, which is a passive restrictive reaction, can be blocked by actual or threatened separation from the mother figure. This may be internalized through overactivation of the parasympathetic nervous system (that system correlated with the passive psychological state), resulting in the release of acetylcholine and bronchial muscle constriction. This is in keeping with the fact that the passive or expiratory phase of respiration is the most markedly affected in asthma. The difficulty with exhalation may also be symbolic of the asthmatic's inability to "let go" of the deep maternal attachments.

From this perspective, asthma, then, revolves around the need to be protected and encompassed. Asthma can thus be called a "suppressed cry for mother's help." Insecurity often underlies this unconscious dependency and, as a result, overcompensation might occur, perhaps assuming the form of competitiveness or excessive striving. This can be seen in children who try to win their mother's approval by outdoing their siblings. Anxiety often accompanies this behavior, which can be explained in part by the decreased supply of oxygen to the brain occurring in an asthmatic attack, and also by the hyperreactive sympathetic system. The sympathetic nervous system and the adrenal glands, which are actually enlarged sympathetic nerve endings, can become exhausted because they attempt to counterbalance the overactive parasympathetic system, which is responsible for producing the acetylcholine that causes the bronchial constriction of asthma. Adrenalin, which is secreted by the adrenals, acts to dilate (open up) the bronchial tubes and at the same time can cause palpitations, sweating, flushing, and a flight of ideas, all of which characterize the anxious state.

Treatment: Physical Level

Nutrition. On the physical level, asthma can be aggravated by imbalances in nutrition, posture, and exercise. From a nutritional perspective, asthma can be minimized by avoidance of mucus-producing foods such as dairy products, glutenous grains (wheat, rye, oats, and barley), refined sugars and flour, starchy fruits like bananas, and red meats. Foods preferred are the other whole grains (corn, millet, buckwheat, and rice), fresh vegetables, fruit, beans and peas, nuts, seeds, and low-fat meats such as fish and chicken. Vitamins considered beneficial in asthma are B, C, E, pantothenic acid, and the mineral manganese. Vitamin C helps to protect the respiratory mucus membrane lining, minimizes allergic tendencies, decreases infection, and counteracts the stress associated with asthma. Vitamin E helps increase oxygenation to cells and Vitamin B complex helps to stabilize the nervous system. Pantothenic acid (one of the B complex) has been reported to stimulate depleted adrenal glands. Manganese has also been reported to decrease the incidence of allergic asthma in patients deficient in that mineral.[1] Herbs that decrease mucus, and are sometimes useful in asthma, are golden seal root, lobelia, slippery elm, and wild cherry bark.

Ayurvedic medicine describes asthma as a combination of excess kaph and vat. This is consistent with modern physiology: a kaph condition is characterized by excess mucus production, and vat refers to imbalance of air, the two principle disturbances in asthma. Ayurveda goes much further, stating that vat potentiates the detrimental effects of

---

[1] Ballentine, *Diet and Nutrition*, p. 242.

excess kaph when the two are combined. Ayurveda further categorizes kaph (mucus) by describing its consistency, odor, color, and taste. These concepts have great therapeutic significance, not only because herbs are prescribed according to the type of kaph, but also because specific foods can be given to counteract and rebalance the effects of vat and kaph. This is accomplished by eating pit foods—those substances that produce fire which can "burn up" excessive mucus and use up the excess air. For example, bajra flour (black millet) and buckwheat flour are especially potent in decreasing mucus and increasing pit. Cooking foods in general increases the fire element. Eating peppercorns fried in clarified butter (ghee) in a fixed daily ratio also increases pit. Adding honey to yogurt tends to cut down on the mucus-producing quality of yogurt.

Cleansing Techniques. Yoga cleansing techniques can be helpful in eliminating excess mucus. In the upper wash, two quarts of salt water are quickly swallowed and then vomited.[2] This practice is done in the morning and helps eliminate mucus from the lungs (mucus is swallowed during the night while one is lying down). The upper wash helps in developing greater control over the vagus nerve, which is in part responsible for the vomiting reflex, and which also mediates the parasympathetic bronchial constriction.

Exercises. The asthmatic individual usually exhibits characteristic problems in body posture. Not uncommon are shoulders hunched forward, accentuated cervical (neck) curves, and tightened chest and back muscles. Specific yoga postures can be used to realign, relax, strengthen, and straighten muscles, bones, joints, and ligaments.

An active exercise program is also advisable to help asthmatics expand their lung reserves, to increase aeration in the lungs where stagnant, trapped air accumulates, and to increase oxygenation to the brain, heart, and other vital

---

[2]The upper wash is not recommended for persons with cardiovascular or kidney problems. See Appendix for further details.

centers. Caution should be taken not to overextend and cause further injury to the areas of tissue damage. Studies suggest that swimming may be particularly beneficial in helping to reduce the frequency and severity of attacks in some asthmatics.[3]

Treatment: Energy Level

Breathing Exercises. For the pranic or energy sheath, yogic breathing exercises and pranayama techniques can help the asthmatic develop control of respiratory movements. Asthma is associated with a prolonged and difficult exhalation. This can lead to increased carbon dioxide build-up and an acidic body condition; each of these conditions can lead to mental and sensory dullness. Listlessness, low energy, and depression can result. Pranayama exercises are helpful because they can increase awareness by improving oxygenation and regulating abnormal respiratory patterns. They can also help to modify and still the parasympathetic nervous system, which will reduce the asthmatic symptomatology.

The flow of pranic energy is also disturbed in asthmatic breathing. Breathing exercises such as the Complete Yogic Breath, diaphragmatic breathing, alternate nostril breathing, and Kapalabhati are of great benefit in asthma because they help to regulate and distribute pranic energy. (See Appendix.)

Three different movements can occur during the process of breathing: the movement of the diaphragm, the movement of the intercostal muscles, and the upward and downward movement of the clavicles (collarbones). This complete, orderly, sequential manner of breathing is not practiced in normal relaxed states, but it can be used to

---

[3]Fitch, et al, "Effects of swimming training on children with asthma," *Archives of Disease in Childhood*, 1976, 51, p. 190.

ment. Because the third chakra is responsible for "fire" production, treatment oriented toward stimulating the gastric or abdominal fire is appropriate. For example, some Ayurvedic or Chinese herbs and foods increase this fire. Certain hatha yoga postures have the same effect. Examples of asanas that are helpful in stimulating the third chakra are the abdominal lift, spinal twist, cobra, and peacock. Techniques of concentration and meditation on the solar plexus can be prescribed to balance third chakra activity and focus awareness and energy.

The fourth chakra is an obvious center for asthma. The heart and lung area is symbolized as the cross (+) or the star of David (✡). It is psychologically associated with love, devotion, and nurturance, all positive attributes of motherhood. It can be inferred, then, that the typical overbearing maternal figure can create tension, constriction, and oppression in the asthmatic child's fourth chakra. This can lead to tightness of the bronchial tubes and shortness of breath. Apathy, or the inability to give love and affection, may also occur if the child fears rejection and withdraws into his own inner, "constricted" world. This withdrawal can be unconsciously expressed through activation of the parasympathetic nervous system, which constricts the bronchial tubes. Fourth chakra weakness is also potentiated by third chakra weakness. It is difficult for the higher center to be balanced if the center below it cannot transfer energy upward.

Many of the therapies already discussed are useful in treating the fourth chakra area. Nutritional observances to decrease mucus production from the lungs and bronchial tubes are important. Many yogic practices can be directed toward opening and balancing the heart chakra. The physical posturing of the asthmatic must first be improved. This includes correcting the forward position of the shoulders and the thoracic spinal kyphosis (hunchback) which serve as body armor to "protect" the asthmatic. Asanas such as the cobra, camel, and bow are helpful to relax tension in the chest. Breathing exercises such as the

Complete Yogic Breath, Kapalabhati and diaphragmatic breathing help expand lung capacity and regulate pranic energy flow. (See Appendix.) Counseling is useful to help the asthmatic express his feelings and thus reduce tension in this area.

Understanding how the psyche and emotions affect the soma helps in both the prevention and treatment of asthma. Guilt can often result from conflicting feelings of dependency and frustration or anger toward an overbearing parent. This can be lessened by expressing these feelings verbally. The psychotherapist helps to reduce the strength of emotions by allowing the patient to transfer dependence onto him and then helping the patient to understand the conflict. Understanding can lead to acceptance of his feelings and then active attempts to change behavioral patterns can be initiated. Analysis of dreams helps the individual to comprehend the inner symbols that reflect unconscious motives and desires. Certain concentration exercises and meditative techniques on the heart center also facilitate greater awareness of this center.

The fifth chakra also is occasionally involved in asthma. This throat chakra is associated with communication and growth. The asthmatic often cannot express his real feelings, which can lead to tension and constriction in the throat area, thereby inhibiting the smooth flow of breath. Asthma, in such a case, might be focused in the upper part of the respiratory conducting system, the upper bronchi, trachea, or larynx. The normally smooth laminar flow of air is impeded by narrowed passageways. Therapy in this instance is directed at opening constricted channels in the throat area.

A Treatment Plan

Mr. D., the patient whose profile was described at the beginning of this chapter, was treated in a multilevel way. The yogic model of the sheaths and the chakras provided a framework for an approach that included the many aspects of his disease.

Nutritionally, he was taken off all dairy products and, after allergy testing for food indicated he was allergic to most gluten-containing grains, he was advised to limit his wheat and oat intake. Vitamins A, C, B-6, and pantothenic acid were also prescribed. A herbal tea combination of ephedra, mullein, calendula, comfrey root, ginger root, licorice root, and pleurisy root was taken three times daily. An aerobic exercise program, which consisted of daily alternation of running and swimming, was undertaken. Breathing exercises that included the Complete Yoga Breath, Kapalabhati, and diaphragmatic breathing were done twice daily, along with progressive relaxation. EMG biofeedback was initiated with a focus on relaxation of the forehead and chest areas, and a visualization was taught in which he imagined his bronchial tubes to be greatly expanded hollow tubes that allowed large volumes of air to enter and exit.

He was slowly weaned off drugs (theophylline and an isoproterenol inhalant) and put on low potency homeopathic remedies which included *Natrum Sulphuricum* for asthma coming on at 4:00-5:00 a.m. or during damp weather, *Arsenicum Album* for asthma occurring between 12:00-2:00 a.m. with associated extreme anxiety, and *Ipecac* for asthma associated with vomiting (for relief of symptoms). Constitutional remedies were given including *Sulphur*, *Thuja*, *Staphysagria*, and high potency *Natrum Sulphuricum*.

Concurrent psychotherapy was begun with special emphasis on working out anger and on dream analysis. The patient slowly began to recognize his repressed frustration and to assert himself with his parents. He was able to redefine important familial boundaries and psychologically to separate from his family. Recurrent dreams of doing poorly on school exams and of losing important possessions, which reflected an inner fear of rejection and failure, began to be replaced by dreams of success. His attitude and self-confidence also improved. Slowly, the intensity of his asthma attacks diminished and subsequent minor bouts of wheezing were easily handled by the appropriate homeopathic remedy. Thus, not only were his symptoms relieved through treatment, but his self-concept and the quality of his life were greatly improved.

13

Ulcers

A fifty-year-old man, R. F., developed a duodenal ulcer after years of excessive belching and heartburn. He is a busy executive who spends long hours at work, worries about corporate finances, and spends little time with his family. He relates having a difficult time showing affection outwardly and often avoids emotional expression by working too hard. In a similar way, his parents always had a difficult time showing or telling him that they loved him. Despite his cool exterior, inwardly he felt insecure and vulnerable. He wished he could be more open, but each time he felt the urge to express himself emotionally he closed off quickly to try to appear calm.

His current illness came on when his business developed financial problems. He felt as though he were a failure, had anxiety attacks, and developed severe ulcer pains. His facade of authority and power was eroded, and he had a strong desire to run away and be nurtured by his family. This conflict of trying to appear outwardly strong while feeling weak inwardly and wanting to withdraw seemed to result in the activation of the parasympathetic-type response and subsequent development of ulcer symptomatology.

With this typical case in mind, we will examine the various aspects of ulcers as they involve physical, emotional, mental, and spiritual factors, and also examine some alternative ways of treatment.

Causes of Ulcers

The acids in the stomach are very powerful, strong enough to dissolve metal. To prevent the acid from eating through the walls of the stomach, a thick, tenacious mucus is produced, which lines the wall and protects the delicate cells from the noxious acid. This mechanism breaks down when too much acid or not enough mucus is produced. As a result, the acid comes in contact with the stomach lining and begins eating its way through. If the process is minimal, it may not be noticed at all or may simply appear as common "heartburn." If allowed to continue, a large crater or even a hole may be produced in the stomach. This is called an ulcer, and is one of the more common manifestations of disease in the gastro-intestinal system.

Gastric ulcers occur in the stomach and duodenal ulcers in the duodenum, the first section of the small intestine. Initially, the only symptom may be a sensation of burning in the stomach, which is relieved by eating, as the food neutralizes stomach acid. If the condition progresses, the ulcer may erode through a blood vessel, and bleeding will then occur. This may show itself either by the vomiting of blood or more commonly by black bowel movements, indicative of digested blood in the stool. Finally, the ulcer can literally erode through the stomach wall. When this occurs, the stomach secretions pass into the abdominal cavity, leading to peritonitis, a potentially fatal condition where the abdominal cavity becomes inflamed and infected.

It is important to understand that an ulcer does not develop overnight. It usually takes weeks, months, or possibly years of gastric malfunction to induce ulcer formation. Certain conditions are known to favor ulcer development: the use of coffee, alcohol, cigarettes, and possibly excess use of refined sugar. Certain drugs like aspirin and cortisone can predispose a person to ulcer development. Psychological factors and stressful situations have long been known to strongly influence stomach function and are a major consideration in the development of ulcer disease.

The stomach is in direct communication with the brain via the autonomic nervous system. Specifically, the vagus nerve (the parasympathetic mediator) as well as sympathetic nerves innervate individual gastric cells. Activation of the vagus nerve signals the stomach to secrete digestive juices and to increase blood circulation to the stomach. When a person looks at a fresh loaf of bread and smells its rich aroma, nerve impulses are sent through a series of neural pathways from the eyes and nose to the hypothalamus, which then relays messages to the vagus nerve and eventually to the stomach to get ready for work. An opposite response might occur if a person walks down a dark street and sees someone coming in the other direction carrying a large stick. Immediately the sympathetic nervous system becomes activated. In this case, the blood vessels of the stomach contract to inhibit blood flow to the stomach so that blood can be redirected to the heart, brain, and skeletal musculature in order to react to the potentially dangerous situation. This is perceived as a knot in the stomach, and if something is eaten at this time, it will not "sit" very well. Thus, the parasympathetic nervous system stimulates digestion and the sympathetic inhibits digestion.

Oversecretion of stomach acid is the result of chronic stimulation by the parasympathetic vagus nerve. One of the more common allopathic approaches to an ulcer which does not respond to milder treatment is to perform a vagotomy, to cut the vagus nerve so that the stomach's normal means of being stimulated by the brain is severed. It should be remembered that the vagus nerve has its origin in the deep recesses of the brain. There are many factors which influence response of the vagus. Besides normal physiologic reflexes that mediate functioning of this nerve, the limbic system, which is the emotional center, as well as the higher or cortical centers of the brain, also have an effect. It is through this mechanism that emotional reactions such as anger or fear can influence the functioning of the gastrointestinal system.

According to psychosomatic medical theory, the basic unresolved psychological issue in ulcer patients is a conflict between the ego's desire to assert itself, to demonstrate its independence, strength, and self-sufficiency, and infantile needs to be nurtured and loved. In such a conflict, if the ego is weak and the infantile needs are strong, the person may choose to deal with the conflict in a passive way by withdrawing from it. However, societal values may view overt withdrawal from conflict as a sign of weakness. Therefore, the person compensates by withdrawing only symbolically, through activation of the parasympathetic nervous system. This system is associated with the activation of passive internal processes such as digestion, leading to gastric acid overstimulation.

Psychologically, the unfulfilled need to gratify feelings of infantile dependency is consistent with the eventual formation of an ulcer. Being fed is the earliest way that the infant is able to resolve his anxiety. The child identifies nourishment with a decrease in stress and with security. For some, this craving for oral gratification persists throughout life, and lighting a cigarette, biting fingernails, or munching on a piece of candy serves as the prime method for dealing with anxiety. The ulcer patient's anxiety is compensated for internally by the unconscious activation of the neurogastric pathways rather than by more conscious external ways.

Thus the need to be loved (the resolution of anxiety) becomes converted into the need to be fed. This wish to be nurtured becomes manifest as an activation of the cells which produce stomach acid. This increase in acid production is the body's way of preparing itself for the nurturing which it desires but is unable to obtain. "In such a situation, the stomach responds continuously as if food were being taken in, or about to be taken in . . . the greater the rejection of every receptive gratification, the greater will be this unconscious 'hunger' for love and help. The patient desires food as a symbol of love and help rather than as satiation of a physiological need."[1]

As in the case of Mr. F., when the typical hard-working executive finds himself in a particularly precarious or stressful situation, the pressure to assert independence and strength may clash with infantile desires to be nurtured, passive, and dependent. One practical solution, at least as far as his unconscious mind is concerned, is to develop an ulcer. This kind of conflict can occur in people from all walks of life. An ulcer creates a situation which permits one to rest, withdraw graciously, and accept comfort and support.

Treatment: Physical Level

Nutrition and Ayurvedic Medicine. According to Ayurveda, the stomach and duodenal area correspond to the primary seat of the dosha pit, or the digestive fire. It is here that the food is burned up and prana is liberated to provide the energy needed to sustain life. If a person experiences burning abdominal pain, the Ayurvedic physician will explain that there is too much pit and will treat the patient to reduce it. This therapeutic approach includes several different treatments. First, the patient is advised to eliminate foods that create excessive quantities of pit, like hot or spicy foods and stimulants such as coffee, tobacco, and alcohol. Raw foods such as nuts and salads would also be eliminated because these foods are very complex structurally and require more pit or digestive fire to be broken down. A diet is prescribed based on foods with a cooling or kaphic effect such as milk and yogurt or other foods such as well-cooked vegetables and grains. Cooked foods are more digestible and stimulate less pit to insure their assimilation.

These dietary recommendations are very similar to the

---

[1]Alexander, *Psychosomatic Medicine*, p. 104.

standard ulcer diet. While the Western physician recommends a diet based on the principle of reducing or neutralizing the effects of the surplus acid, the Ayurvedic physician is simply trying to eliminate excess pit. One point of interest here is that drinking milk has classically been known to reduce ulcer pain, yet the exact reason for this has escaped Western physiologists. Claims that milk effectively neutralizes acid or "coats the stomach" have not been substantiated. However, in Ayurvedic terms the reasoning is simple. Milk is a kaphic food and therefore stimulates mucus production. This excess mucus provides an increased protective barrier against the acid and therefore reduces inflammation and pain.

Ayurveda also takes into account the psychological factors that increase pit, such as anger. To be "red with rage" may not only represent a psychological attitude, but also will manifest in the body as increased anger or pit. People with fiery temperaments have too much pit and therefore may have too much fire stored in the "pit center" or solar plexus. To decrease this quantity of pit and reduce the excess fire, the Ayurvedic physician may not only prescribe a diet, but will often give the patient a herb or perhaps a mantra or meditative practice. The use of meditation and relaxation to treat ulcers, although a relatively new approach in the West, has been used traditionally in the East.

Exercise. The establishment of a consistent, progressive program of physical activity such as jogging can be helpful in ulcer disease. Jogging or other aerobic exercises can be an outlet for the release of anxiety that has taken the form of muscular tension. In view of the proposed psychosomatic model and the role of anxiety in the genesis of ulcers, the relaxation of muscle tension and the sense of well-being associated with vigorous exercise are very important.

Hatha yoga's role in ulcer disease relates to the understanding that the student develops concerning the relationship between mental and physical tension. General muscular tension reflects mental unrest, and this tension becomes "stored" in the muscles that line the digestive tract.

Release of skeletal muscular tension facilitates relaxation of muscles that line internal organs. (See Chapter 7.)

Treatment: Energy Level

Breathing Exercises. Diaphragmatic breathing is beneficial in the treatment of ulcers. Because of the close relationship between the breath and the emotions, breathing exercises help to decrease the anxiety associated with the conflict of ego-strength. The chronic activation of the parasympathetic nervous system associated with ulcers can be relaxed by breathing exercises. Since breath provides a bridge between the voluntary and autonomic nervous systems, the breath can be a tool for consciously regulating autonomic nervous system activity.

Biofeedback. Biofeedback training helps the person become aware of tension and what it feels like to be relaxed. The EMG applied to the muscles of the abdominal wall may accurately reflect tension in the stomach and intestines. Through the use of the temperature trainer, the ulcer patient can learn relaxation and thus begin to regulate the autonomic nervous system. Relaxation is a help in healing ulcers.

Homeopathy and Yoga. *Arsenicum Album* and *Nux Vomica* are two of many homeopathic remedies which are very effective in treating ulcers. *Arsenicum Album* is characteristically prescribed for an individual who is subject to great fearfulness, restlessness, and insecurity. There is a "morbid dread of friends and family deserting them," of being left alone, perhaps to die. Physically there is profuse diarrhea, usually burning the rectum. There are burning discharges from most of the body orifices including the eyes, ears, nose, bladder, lungs, vagina, uterus, and skin.

The reader will notice that the remedy *Arsenicum Album* is found under two disease discussions: asthma and ulcers. It is one of several remedies called polychrests which are frequently used in clinical practice. *Arsenicum* is a remedy that affects almost all organ systems, and it is a good example of a remedy that can be used to treat many diverse problems. We have indicated that a certain emotional and psychological type needs *Arsenicum* irrespective of the category of disease, which illustrates that it is the person who is treated, and not just the illness.

From a yogic standpoint, the first and the third chakras are affected in the *Arsenicum* state. In the yogic model, the first chakra is associated physiologically with the act of elimination, and some practitioners link it psychologically with security and possession. Security, the desire for ego-survival, is the most primitive of all acts. All organisms, from the most primitive protozoan to man, have this instinct. It is so inbred into our being that it need not interfere with our conscious processes. A healthy balance of energy at the first chakra is very important because it can establish a secure and protected feeling in the individual, which provides the foundation and strength upon which to build a healthy body and mind. Although egotism is eventually overcome, a strong, intact ego and sense of self are mandatory for the balanced functioning of the higher chakras. If the first chakra energy is dissipated, then a person's psychophysiological matrix will be weakened, as may be manifested by chronic constipation or diarrhea on the physical level or anxiety and paranoia on the mental level.

In the *Arsenicum* state of pathology, this insecurity and anxiety is compensated for by the need to control everyone and everything that may affect one's security. This resultant struggle for control or power may become evident as imbalances in the third chakra.

In yoga psychology, an ulcer represents an imbalance in the third chakra (solar plexus), located at the stomach area, around the navel. This chakra, situated in the center of the digestive tract, is associated with metabolism of food and is related to oral psychological attitudes. Imbalances manifest here as digestive or metabolic difficulties such as ulcers or diabetes mellitus.

The yoga model implies that power conflicts are most

likely to develop problems around the third chakra area, such as gastric illnesses. Individuals with difficulties at this area present themselves in one of two ways. Either they are overly self-assertive, characterized by the go-getting, hard-driving, nobody-is-going-to-get-in-my-way businessman, or the opposite, passive, disgruntled, silently disenchanted, and feeling like "the whole world is picking on me." In either case, the common denominator is the "me against them" attitude. Both types are often classified as characteristic ulcer personalities.

The excessive burning pains, which are characteristic symptoms of the *Arsenicum* picture, indicate that the third chakra or solar plexus area is overactive. The inner heat increases in intensity, creating burning discharges and ulcerations of the mucus membranes, especially along the upper respiratory passages and in the solar plexus areas itself. Yoga philosophy would say that samana, the prana responsible for digestion and metabolism, is hyperfunctional. Because the inner fires burn in an exaggerated way, the fuel is quickly consumed, leaving the system devoid of the heating element. The feet and hands get frigid and blue, the blood vessels feel "as though ice water runs through them," and the perspiration becomes cold. These latter symptoms are definitive hallmarks of the homeopathic remedy *Arsenicum Album*.

Nux Vomica is another remedy that is frequently indicated in the treatment of ulcers. The patient for whom *Nux* is suitable is often the overly ambitious person who is interested primarily in self-fulfillment. He is frequently selfish, caring only for his needs, often overlooking or abusing the emotions and requirements of others. The strong need of the *Nux* personality to be nurtured and satisfied can be inferred from his marked predilection for overindulgence in food, drink, and stimulants. Interestingly, the *Nux* patient is often the typical ulcer patient, like Mr. F., the case described earlier, whose conflict leads to difficulties in digestion (nausea, vomiting, belching) and ulcer formation, all third chakra symptoms. As in the *Arsenicum* type patient, the conflicts at the third chakra cause the system to create an overabundance of heat. This helps explain the *Nux Vomica* symptoms of the "skin feeling hot, especially during fevers, despite an inner feeling of coldness" and "a great need to be covered up."

Treatment: Mental Level

Meditation and/or psychotherapy are of paramount importance in holistic medicine therapeutics to help prevent or heal ulcers. The suffering individual needs to understand psychological disturbances that underlie his gastric problems. By becoming aware of emotional conflicts that are associated with ulcer disease, a person can actually transform his discomfort into a learning experience. Awareness is the first step, and this is followed by learning to integrate the knowledge gained through self-awareness into practical methods to eliminate the digestive problems.

Enhanced awareness of how physical habits, personality traits, and emotional conflicts lead to disorders of the digestive system can result from both psychotherapy and meditation. Through slow, methodic psychological insight, energy is redirected from creating abnormal physiologic conditions like ulcers and lower bowel disorders and is liberated to help better integrate body, mind, and spirit.

A Treatment Plan

R. F., the case with which this chapter began, received treatment on various levels. Dietary management was integral in controlling his ulcer disease. Alcohol, tobacco, coffee, and spicy foods were eliminated because of their irritating qualities. The patient was placed on a diet of lean meat including fish, poultry, and veal. He was instructed to eat frequent small meals and to avoid raw food because it could irritate the ulcer. Cooked vegetables and cooked whole grains and yogurt were to be eaten. Slowly chewing almonds was helpful in decreasing hyperacidic symptoms.

The patient was instructed in diaphragmatic breathing and relaxation to help him reduce anxiety and balance his overactive nervous system. He also began an exercise program which consisted of twenty minutes of brisk walking everyday. Biofeedback training with the EMG was used over the forehead and abdominal muscles to help him understand how muscle tension is associated with painful ulcer episodes.

Within three months after making these changes, he was virtually without symptoms of digestive problems—for the first time in years. During this three month period he began psychotherapy, which helped him substantially with identifying feelings of fear and sadness and learning to express these feelings more directly with his family and friends. Thus, coping with his illness started this patient on a path toward self-knowledge and a fuller, more rewarding life.

14

Hyperthyroidism

Mrs. B. is a fifty-year-old woman who developed symptoms of hyperthyroidism, including an enlarged thyroid, fatigue, agitated depression, palpitation, weight loss, increased perspiration, and hair loss. Although she had felt fatigue for approximately one year prior to onset of the disease, the hyperthyroidism coincided with severe marital quarreling. She said that she was feeling very incompetent, insecure, and continuously feared being abandoned by her second husband, who was sixteen years younger than herself. She had tended to dominate their relationship and in a sense "mother" her spouse. When he began to resist this behavior and assert his independence, her symptoms began. It appears that her defense against feelings of insecurity and rejection was to assume a role of controlling her husband's life, since she couldn't control her own life.

This patient related that she was dominated by her own mother and said after spending a week with her that "I have to stick up for myself." Never having felt love from her mother, she married at an early age in an attempt to attain security by becoming a mother herself. She could never express her negative or angry feelings to her mother and would feel tightness in her throat. Her excessive passivity towards her mother was transferred to her growing children, whom she smothered in an overcompensating way to give them what she never had. Her children couldn't handle this passive-aggressiveness and eventually left home and avoided further communication.

As with the other cases discussed in this section, this woman was treated with a multilevel approach. After examining various aspects of hyperthyroidism, we will present a treatment plan that was successful in curing her condition and making her more whole as a person.

Causes of Hyperthyroidism

The thyroid gland is an endocrine organ divided into three major parts: the right lobe, the left lobe, and the isthmus, which interconnects the lobes. It is located alongside and slightly below the laryngeal protrusion (Adam's apple). The major function of the thyroid gland is to produce an iodine-containing hormone called thyroxin, which has many essential roles in maintaining health.

Thyroxin is responsible for controlling the rate of body metabolism and is needed for normal physical and mental growth. Deficiencies in this hormone lead to premature cessation of bone growth and mental retardation. Overproduction leads to extreme weight loss, anxiety, and nervousness. Thyroxin's role in reproduction, development, and maturation is well established. Levels of thyroxin rise in pregnancy, and this hormone is responsible for stimulating genital duct formation in the male. Underactivity of the thyroid leads to decreased sex drive, miscarriage, and sterility.

On the emotional and mental levels, thyroxin exerts important influences, as the qualities of alertness, sensitivity, and clarity of thought are dependent upon adequate supplies. Deficiency causes mental sluggishness, while excess thyroxin augments sensitivity and awareness to the point where the person can become anxious, hypersensitive, and suffer from insomnia.

Thyroid hormone functioning increases when there are longstanding stresses on the body or mind such as occur in pregnancy. It acts in a similar way to the sympathetic nervous system hormone adrenalin, although the latter hormone is generally released during acute, sudden stress, while thyroxin is secreted during chronic stress states. The association between thyroxin and adrenalin is also seen in people with hyperactive thyroid glands who overreact to small amounts of adrenaline.

The anterior pituitary in the brain secretes a hormone called thyroid stimulating hormone (TSH) which causes the thyroid to produce more thyroxin. TSH in turn is controlled by a substance made in the hypothalamus called thyroid releasing factor (TRF). TRF may be affected by higher brain centers such as the cerebral cortex and limbic system. This may provide the explanation of how thoughts and emotions can affect the production of thyroxin. Thyroxin itself has a negative feedback on both TSH and TRF, which means that when blood levels of thyroxin are high enough, thyroxin will signal directly to the pituitary and hypothalamus to stop secretion of their hormones.

Hyperthyroidism, also called thyrotoxicosis, is characterized by overproduction of thyroid hormone. Symptoms associated with this illness reflect an exaggeration of all the normal functions controlled by thyroid hormone. Among these are anxiety, extreme restlessness, weight loss despite increased appetite, sweating, hair loss, palpitations of the heart, and bulging of the eyes (exopthalamus). These symptoms are quite similar to those found in the anxiety-stress syndrome of the sympathetic nervous system.

There are several common causes for hyperthyroidism, which include: (1) overactive nodules of thyroid tissue or tumors of the thyroid; and (2) generally enlarged and overactive thyroid gland. The thyroid gland can also be enlarged when it is underactive. Iodine is important in the synthesis of thyroxin, and iodine deficiency occurs in certain locales where iodine levels in the soil are low, such as in the Great Lake areas where the glaciers leached the iodine out as they retreated toward the Arctic. In such cases, the gland works harder and enlarges in an attempt to produce enough functional thyroxin to provide for the body's needs. Here the thyroid gland is hypofunctional because of missing iodine.

According to psychoanalytic theory, the most frequent conflict that typifies the hyperthyroid patient is difficulty in exchanging the roles of being nurtured and nurturing others. At the root of this conflict is an intense insecurity characterized by a fear of death or loss of maternal love accompanied by worry about taking over the burden of motherhood. It is not surprising that the great majority of hyperthyroid patients are female. These people psychologically struggle against this insecurity by trying to master it through controlling external emotions or increasing their sense of responsibility. The first psychological defense, that of not expressing emotions, leads to tension and rigidity in the throat and larynx area and results in a chronic inability to communicate. The second defense is curious. In an effort to overcome the anxiety or fear of the loss of maternal support, the person may compulsively try to master that which is feared. A "pseudo-maturity" develops, resulting in an attempt to assume a parental role in order to decrease the discomforting feelings of insecurity. This self-reliance, however, is hollow because such a person is not internally ready for this role.

A common way to combat the fear of maternal loss is by becoming pregnant or by becoming a mother figure to siblings. Becoming pregnant combats the fear of death through the act of bringing another life into the world, and it also counteracts the fear of losing the mother by "becoming a mother." Being motherly to siblings can bring about vicarious gratifications of dependency needs.

Feelings of insecurity often originate in early childhood upon experiencing parental death or divorce, maternal indifference, or from actually witnessing the death of someone close. A long-term facade of maturity may then be assumed to disguise or conceal the feelings of insecurity or nurturance needs. As long as the defense (hyperactivity, pregnancy, etc.) remains intact, the individual may continue to live normally within the pseudomature role. However, when stressful situations such as illness or miscarriage threaten these defenses, or when a child leaves home, underlying anxiety surfaces. This creates more stress on the part of the maturation system associated with the thyroid gland, already under chronic activation since childhood because of the constant demands for accelerated maturity. When the vicissitudes of life overwhelm the struggle to control anxiety and dependency needs through premature self-reliance roles, hyperthyroidism can result.

According to the yogic model, physical, mental, and spiritual issues relating to the fifth chakra predominate when the thyroid becomes diseased. This chakra is said to be associated with the ability to be nurtured, feelings of trust, communicative functions, and the creative potential.

Being nurtured involves the ability to be receptive, open, and trusting toward the provider. The child receives sustenance from the mother, while the adult obtains nurturance from the external environment, interpersonal relationships, and the inner self. Nurturance can be in the form of food, material goods, or emotional support. Guidance from one's conscience or inner feelings is also a form of nurturance.

According to this theory, the giving of nurturance is a concern of the fourth chakra, which involves feeling love for others. Receiving nurturance is, in a sense, a higher capacity than giving it, and the ability to accept love and guidance from within and without is a function of an integrated, balanced, well-focused fifth chakra. Trust is also a quality of the fifth chakra. When a person fears rejection, as happens in hyperthyroidism, there is a tendency to mistrust others and fear of being hurt or abandoned. This is in accordance with the psychosomatic model, where the most prominent emotional conflicts associated with hyperthyroidism are the fear of maternal loss or rejection and feelings of insecurity. There is an overpowering fear that one will not be taken care of or nurtured.

The ability to communicate with clarity is also an important aspect of the fifth chakra, since the larynx and voice box, essential for speech and verbal expression, are located in the throat area. The physical counterparts of emotional shock or anxiety which manifest in the throat area are the feeling of "a lump in the throat" and a tight or constricted sensation in the throat. People who have tension in this area often "lose their voice" or "can't find the right words to express themselves." Hyperthyroid people often have similar blocks, either because of a severe emotional shock which precipitates the hyperthyroidism, or because of chronic repression of fears and anxieties.

Creativity, which is said to be characteristic of a focused and well-balanced fifth chakra, involves the ability to tap into one's inner potential. Deep within the unconscious lie hidden abilities, knowledge, and sources of great inspiration. Insights gained from this vast reservoir allow individuals to express themselves creatively. The results can be seen in great achievements in art, music, or literature and also in skill and productiveness in any endeavor that involves precision or ingenuity. To experience truly creative inspiration, the conscious mind and egoistic tendencies must not be allowed to interfere with the fresh, pure aspects of the unconscious mind. The individual must be open to receive nurturance from within and to be a channel and receptacle for the finer secrets of life that emerge from deep inside the creative centers.

The creative urge, an expression of the fifth chakra, is blocked in persons with thyroid problems. The characteristic defense of the hyperthyroid individual are psychological barriers which inhibit the inner flow of creative thought and understanding. A person who utilizes various defenses in his relationships is employing conscious effort which requires great amounts of energy. The unconscious potential is kept in abeyance by the hyperactivity of conscious preoccupation.

Creativity leads to evolution and growth of consciousness. As a person integrates more and more of the unknown with the known, the universe becomes more understandable and controllable. The fifth chakra is the steppingstone to the two highest chakras, and it is at the highest centers of consciousness that integration leads to true intuitive knowledge and expanded awareness.

Treatment: Physical Level

Treatment oriented toward the fifth chakra includes postures that stimulate the throat area: the shoulder stand, fish, bridge, and general stretching exercises for the neck and shoulders. The lion's pose is also helpful if practiced twice a day.

The upper wash, in which water is swallowed and then regurgitated (see Appendix), not only helps rid the system of excess mucus but is also beneficial in several other ways. Tension in the throat is often associated with the fear of letting go of emotions. Vomiting, an act of letting go or releasing, can relieve these physical and emotional tensions. Individuals with problems in the throat area often fear vomiting, and the upper wash can help to gradually eliminate this fear.

Treatment: Energy Level

Breathing Exercises. Breathing exercises are very valuable in thyroid disease, especially bhramari and ujjaya, which directly stimulate the thyroid area. Diaphragmatic breathing accompanied by relaxation techniques helps to re-establish a smooth air flow through tightened throat areas where the thyroid gland is situated. Kapalabhati, through its more vigorous vibrational stimulation, can positively affect the thyroid gland functioning. (See Appendix.)

Homeopathy. There are several homeopathic remedies

that can help to cure hyperthyroidism. By acting on the vital force, which in this case is in a state of chronic overstimulation, the similar remedy helps to re-establish physiologic balance and to catalyze psychological growth. After taking the homeopathic remedy, the patient carefully notes changing symptoms and emotional attitudes that affect the entire system. In working with the physician, he learns to recognize personality patterns and underlying conflicts that may predispose him to the thyrotoxic condition. Recognition of these conflicts is a most important step in changing habits and psychological attitudes. More mature methods of handling problems can be substituted for infantile coping and defense mechanisms.

Natrum Muriaticum (sodium chloride) is a primary homeopathic remedy to consider in the hyperthyroid condition. This substance is interesting, both from a physiologic viewpoint and from a psychological-symbolic perspective. On the physical level, sodium chloride helps to maintain normal blood volume and blood pressure. Most molecular particles depend on a normal concentration of sodium in water to facilitate their free movement through the body's tissues. In the Eastern tradition of Ayurvedic medicine, salt is considerd a very powerful stimulant, and one is cautioned to use it with discrimination. Chinese medicine views salt as a yang substance which, if taken in excess, can lead to yang symptoms such as aggression and heat production.

In the West, sodium chloride (table salt) is overused because artificial foods are devoid of taste, and salt brings out added flavor. Also, because salt is a stimulant, it is used to provide a physical and mental lift. In the U.S. salt is not only added in the preparation of foods but is also used as a preservative in most prepackaged foods. The result is an intake of as much as fifty to a hundred times the daily requirement. Because of this, symptoms can occur that mimic those of thyrotoxicosis, such as anxiety, palpitations, and sweating.

From a psychological standpoint, *Natrum Mur* is symbolic of the ocean, since salt is the main substance found within the sea. Because the earliest plant and animal life began in the ocean, it represents the primordial pool from which all life stems. It is symbolically equivalent to the mother archetype. The ocean, like the mother, is the giver of life. The watersac (amniotic fluid) that bathes the growing embryo in the womb is comprised of salt water and is another instance of the relationship between the ocean, the origin of life, and the mother. Emotional problems centered around the mother figure, typical of thyroid hyperactivity, offer a further analogy. It is interesting that imbalances which may play a key role in thyroid disease call for the homeopathic remedy *Natrum Mur*. Because the remedy acts on the subtle energy level, a psychological analogy such as this is interesting and relevant.

The other remedy which is often used and which typifies the overactive state of thyrotoxicosis is *Iodine*. We have seen that *Iodine* is important in the synthesis of thyroxin and imbalances in its metabolism greatly affect the functioning of the thyroid gland. When indicated, iodine used homeopathically helps to balance the overactive thyroid gland. It is interesting to note that iodine is added to table salt to be sold in iodine-deficient locales.

Hypothyroidism, or low thyroxin production, is characterized by sluggish metabolism, slow heart rate, and deficient mentation. The remedy most closely associated with these symptoms is *Calcarea Carbonica*, which is calcium carbonate derived from the oyster shell. Symbology applies here, too. The oyster, which lives in the salty sea, is surrounded by a firm, rigid shell that protects the animal but also restricts it. Thus, *Calcarea Carbonica* represents restrictive, narrowed, and slowed down phenomena in the sea. Its use in hypothyroidism becomes obvious. The oyster withdraws from danger and the outer environment by becoming enclosed within its protective shell. It is interesting that hypothyroidism seems to occur most often in persons who are overprotective of themselves and their families and who tend to withdraw from conflict.

The remedy *Natrum Mur* was earlier seen to be symbolically analogous to and therapeutically useful in conditions that are characteristically hyperfunctional and overactive. This is equivalent to the sympathetic nervous system response pattern. *Calcarea Carb*, on the other hand, is associated with restrictive, passive, withdrawing qualities, and thus is analogous to the parasympathetic nervous system type response.

Treatment: Mental Level

Learning to verbalize internal problems through psychotherapy often helps to release throat tension. Free verbal expression of locked-in feelings and thoughts can help open up the throat chakra. Similarly, crying, laughing, and singing may provide an outlet for tension, making possible relaxation of the throat. Techniques of concentration and meditation on the throat help to focus awareness and energy. They will decrease the tendency toward dissipation of energy and help to control and direct it for more creative purposes.

A Treatment Plan

Holistic treatment for Mrs. B., our typical hyperthyroidism case, included decreasing excessively stimulating foods such as salt, spices, and sweets, as these tend to stimulate an already hyperfunctioning thyroid condition. Spending much time in relaxation and meditation and walking only slowly were suggested to help cultivate a quiet state of mind and body. Biofeedback was initiated, with special emphasis on learning to relax the areas over the thyroid gland. To further promote a calm state, she was instructed to focus her attention on the thyroid area (fifth chakra) and visualize the full moon in a blue sky. Homeopathic remedies were successful, so that drugs and radiation therapy could be avoided. *Natrum Muriaticum*, *Calcarea Iodatum*, and *Medorrhinum* were among the more important remedies used.

Psychotherapy was helpful. Since this patient was not inclined to remember her dreams or take an interest in early childhood experiences, problem solving was employed mostly rather than any kind of intensive analysis. However, during treatment, Mrs. B. gradually became aware of her immature behavior patterns and underlying fears. She began to assume a more realistic role as wife and to let go of her controlling characteristics. She became more independent and actually got a job, for the first time in her life. As a consequence, communication with her husband improved and the marriage became relatively harmonious. She came to understand and accept why her children avoided contact with her. In essence, she became a mature woman,

15

Lower Bowel Disorders

L. W. is a twenty-eight-year-old woman who, six months prior to being seen, had developed daily episodes of lower abdominal cramping pain, flatulence, and diarrhea. These symptoms began when the patient started a job as a store manager. She stated that she never felt confident about functioning in positions of authority, although she always sought these types of jobs. She tried to push these feelings aside and prove herself capable of this new challenge. As demands by her management superiors increased, and as problem-solving with the people she was supervising was proving ineffective, the patient's level of anxiety about failing became stronger and the above symptoms began. Prior to this, similar situations resulted in anxiety felt in the pit of the stomach and occasional episodes of painless diarrhea. The patient saw a physician after the cramping pain and diarrhea had persisted for one month. A barium enema examination of the colon was performed, and the patient was diagnosed as having spastic colitis. A medication to block the overactivity of the parasympathetic nervous system was prescribed, but she experienced only minimal relief of her symptoms. She continued with her job, and her symptoms varied according to the amount of stress she experienced in her work.

From the point of view of psychosomatic medicine, this person showed a pattern of symptom development which corresponds with psychological characteristics often seen in colitis patients: an underlying insecurity concerning basic self-confidence and ability to perform. When she was stressed by this new job beyond her ability to cope, rather than withdrawing by quitting, she persevered on a conscious level. But the urge to withdraw was expressed symbolically by activation of the parasympathetic nervous system, and the symptoms of colitis ensued.

Causes of Constipation and Diarrhea

Bowel motility (peristaltic movement) is controlled by the parasympathetic system, and under normal situations this process occurs in a controlled, gentle, and synchronistic way. *Diarrhea* can occur when parasympathetic overactivation increases bowel motility, rushing food through the small intestine and colon before it can be adequately digested and absorbed. Conversely, when one is in a state of fear, the sympathetic system becomes activated and blood is rechanneled to the organs necessary for immediate survival, such as the muscles and brain. Activity is inhibited in the other organ systems, such as the urinary and digestive, which are not critical for immediate survival. In order to facilitate the relative slowdown in the function of these two systems, a set of reflexes is triggered which cause the bladder to empty and the bowels to evacuate. The sympathetic system causes the rectal sphinctors to relax and the peristaltic and absorbing activities of the bowel to stop. Thus, an underabsorbed, watery stool moves quickly through and out the flaccid large intestine. In acute conditions, fear can cause a child or an animal to defecate or urinate uncontrollably. If a person is in a chronic state of fear or anxiety, a condition of chronic or frequent defecation (diarrhea) will occur. Thus, diarrhea can be due to overactivity of either the parasympathetic or sympathetic nervous systems.

Two common causes of chronic diarrhea are spastic and ulcerative colitis. Diarrhea associated with spasms of the colon but without observable changes in the colon is called spastic colitis. Ulcerative colitis is a more severe form of colitis in which the walls of the colon are covered with tiny ulcers which often ooze blood, leading to painful, bloody evacuations. There are other illnesses which are associated with chronic diarrhea, but ulcerative and spastic colitis are the most frequent causes. Our discussion will be limited to their consideration.

According to the psychosomatic medical theory, individuals suffering from ulcerative or spastic colitis often demonstrate a typical conflict centering in their strong demanding (oral-aggressive) and receptive wishes. These people try to compensate for dependent and receptive wishes by giving in exchange. They want to compensate for all those things which they want to receive or take away from others. This often takes the form of worry about certain duties and obligations, the need to give money or support others, and the urge to exert effort through work. For such reasons, the patient is often described as being overly conscientious. At the same time, however, this person has a violent reluctance to exert himself, to engage in systematic work, or to fulfill those obligations to which he feels emotionally compelled. The patient may become dependent on others, but wants to do something to compensate for all that he receives. Instead of real accomplishment, the patient satisfies his conscience with this infantile form of gift—the intestinal content. This substitute for real accomplishment is obviously a regressive and passive action. This response is mediated by overactivation of the parasympathetic nervous system. Essentially then, certain types of chronic diarrhea are the somatic manifestation of a basic lack of self-confidence. The disease is the outward expression of the act of giving to compensate for unconscious feelings of insecurity.

Constipation, another affliction of modern man, is a condition in which the stool remains in the colon too long and becomes dessicated and hardened. This creates a wide variety of symptoms, including vague feelings of discomfort or bloating, headache, nausea and vomiting, and, in the most extreme cases, results in fecal impaction and blockage of the colon. Chronic constipation can often lead to such conditions as diverticulosis (an outpocketing of the colon wall) and hemorrhoids (a condition where the veins around the anus become dilated). In either case, it is the increased pressure created by straining to pass the hardened stool which can lead to the problem.

People suffering with psychogenic constipation often feel rejected and are pessimistic and distrust others. They feel that they cannot expect much from anyone and feel little need to give. The retention of feces provides a feeling of well-being or security. It is for this reason that some individuals, despite a high fiber diet and enough water and exercise, may still be troubled with constipation.

From a yogic perspective, these people exhibit a conflict in the first chakra, which deals physiologically with the act of elimination, and psychologically with security and possession. Disturbance in this chakra threatens the instinct for survival and may manifest as paranoia. Weakness of the first chakra can also manifest as chronic *diarrhea*, a physical representation of insecurity on the mental-emotional level.

In both cases, there is a passive response according to psychoanalytic theory, but in constipation the psychological issues are fear of rejection with consequent selfishness (the person tries to possess that which he fears losing). Inability to give of one's self is manifested on the physical level as tightness of the rectum and retention of stool. Chronic diarrhea reflects a more integrated ego where the person feels secure enough at least to attempt to give, even if in an infantile way. People with chronic colitis are insecure but are not as self-oriented as those with severe chronic constipation. Thus, in the yoga system, this would be an example of a higher degree of development within an individual chakra as well as an involvement of higher chakras, such as the second if related to sexual insecurity, or the third if related to feelings of inadequacy resulting from issues of power.

Yoga philosophy calls the energy that is responsible for elimination *apana*. This is analogous to the dosha *vat*. In healthy individuals the vat or air moves in a downward direction, but occasionally, things go awry and the vat begins to move upwards. This condition causes problems that may manifest in a number of ways. Constipation will result, as it is the normal downward force of vat which supplies the energy movement of the stool.

Headaches are also a common symptom associated with constipation. No good reason for this relationship has been offered in orthodox medicine, other than the possibility that in the retained stool there are metabolic wastes that irritate nervous tissues in the brain. However, according to Ayurveda headaches can be expected as the vat moves upward and fills the head, and the increased "air" pressure causes pain in the cerebral area. In order to correct this situation, an enema may be prescribed to stimulate a reversal of this flow of vat. As vat again begins to flow downward, the constipation often is relieved and the headache ameliorated.

Flatus (colonic air) is a manifestation of excessive vat, as is diarrhea. The cause may be secondary to diet, e.g., eating predominantly vattic foods like beans, or to a vattic mental state. Treatment should be designed to rebalance the doshas, using a combination of diet, medicines, or meditative exercises.

Treatment: Physical Level

Although constipation may be due to psychogenic causes, in many instances it may also be due to poor nutrition and lack of exercise. It has been noted that the average transit time required for stool to pass through the large bowel varies tremendously according to the quantity of fiber consumed. African tribesmen, who consume large quantities of fiber, have voluminous stools with a transit time of approximately twelve to twenty-four hours. Europeans and Americans, on the other hand, with their highly refined and processed diets, tend to have smaller stools and a transit time of up to seventy-two hours. In an effort to compensate for the lack of fiber, Americans substitute large quantities of bran or other bulk agents. This is only a symptomatic approach. The problem is not a bran deficiency, but a fiber deficiency. Bran is a type of fiber, but it is harsh and can irritate the delicate bowel lining.[1] What is needed is a more natural diet consisting of foods high in natural fiber, such as fruits and vegetables, and especially whole grains and legumes. Since these latter two are often absent in the average diet, it should come as no surprise that many people find themselves constipated.

Other dietary measures are also helpful in treating constipation. In Ayurvedic medicine, psyllium seed husks are prescribed to prevent and treat the disorder. These husks have a gelatinous consistency and, unlike bran, are not irritative but have a gentle action. Since they are indigestible, they provide more than adequate quantities of fiber to aid in elimination. Also effective is drinking a glass of hot water to which have been added the juice from half a lemon, a pinch of salt, and honey to taste. This traditional folk remedy is a very effective natural laxative and is very mild. The use of prune juice, coffee, milk of magnesia, or other strong laxatives is not recommended, since they weaken the body's own ability to eliminate and tend to make the system chronically dependent on their use. Avoiding excessive quantities of dairy products, especially cheese, can also be helpful.

The second important factor in preventing constipation is exercise. Few joggers complain of constipation because the

---

[1]Horace W. Davenport, *Physiology of the Digestive Tract* (Chicago: Year Book Medical Publications, 1982), p. 255.

continuous jostling of the colon stimulates its contraction. Performing certain hatha yoga exercises such as the stomach lift, plow, and knee to chest positions has a gentle massaging affect on the colon and aids in elimination. The biomechanisms of elimination can also be facilitated by squatting. The Western style toilet seat, although aesthetically appealing, is not very functional. A person familiar with the squatting style of toilet used in the East or who has defecated in the woods, will attest to the increased efficiency. Squatting is not only an effective way to decrease the amount of straining required, but it can prevent and alleviate hemorrhoids.

There are many factors which can cause diarrhea. In acute cases it may be due to ingestion of certain foods, micro-organisms, or toxins which the body rejects and attempts to throw off. Acute diarrhea most commonly occurs in conjunction with acute viral intestinal infection. Usually in these cases the process is self-limiting, and a diet of clear liquids or pureed carrot soup will correct the problem.

The chronic diarrhea of ulcerative or spastic colitis is a more complex treatment problem. Dietary guidelines for treating these conditions has significantly changed over the years. In general, nuts, raw fruit and vegetables, uncooked grains, bran, and other foods with heavy roughage should be avoided. Cooked whole grains and cooked vegetables, previously prohibited to patients with chronic diarrhea, are now considered by many physicians to be acceptable and even helpful, the feeling being that the fiber in these foods may act as bulk agents, helping to hold the stool together. Yogurt may help provide a favorable environment for repopulation of the colon with bacteria which may have been lost with frequent diarrhea. Tofu is an excellent source of nonirritating, easily digestible, high quality protein. Stewed and peeled apples are helpful especially since apples contain pectin which helps form the stool. Citrus fruit is very yin, according to Chinese medicine, and should be avoided in this yin condition of chronic watery stools. Cooked whole grains and cooked vegetables are yang and thus can help to balance this condition.

Active exercise would be beneficial in the treatment of the chronic diarrhea of spastic or ulcerative colitis. Relaxation of mind and body afforded by movement would be helpful in minimizing the discharge of tension through the autonomic nervous system. Hatha yoga can be beneficial for the same reasons by helping to reduce internal and external body tension, as well as promoting calm and relaxation. Hatha postures can be performed to promote specific results.

For example, for diarrhea postures should be held for longer periods to keep the abdominal contents relatively stationary. Constipation, on the other hand, would be better treated by repeating the posture in rapid succession to stimulate the sluggish digestive organs. The abdominal lift might be more beneficial when the bowel movements are loose, while agni sara, a variation of the stomach lift, would help constipation. The latter exercise involves quick movements of the abdominal muscles in and out, while the breath is being held in the exhalation phase.

Treatment: Energy Level

We have seen that the psychosomatic medical model elucidates how intimately the autonomic nervous system is tied with lower bowel disorders as well as with ulcers. Because the breath links the mind and body, as well as serving to bring about balance between the parasympathetic and sympathetic parts of the autonomic nervous system, exercises that are focused on creating smooth, rhythmic, effortless breathing patterns are essential for an individual's total health.

By focusing attention on the solar plexus (third chakra) area while breathing with the diaphragm, greater balance is brought to the sympathetic and parasympathetic nervous systems which innervate this nerve plexus. Since the sympathetic nervous system originates from the back-chest area, the sympathetic part of the ANS is quieted by not stimulating these areas with chest breathing. The emotional responses to psychological conflicts are also brought under greater conscious control by diaphragmatic breathing coupled with a relaxation technique. Thus the emotional conflicts are minimized or eliminated, and the physiological system is better balanced. These practices, along with a coordinated nutritional, exercise, and meditative or psychological program, can lead to resolution of these lower bowel disorders.

Homeopathy. Lycopodium (club moss) is a remedy which typifies the symptoms that a person has with lower bowel disorders, especially those people who have chronic constipation alternating with loose stools. A person who needs *Lycopodium* is full of trapped gas, often developing flatus while eating. As is typical of the constipated individual described in psychoanalytic theory, a person needing *Lycopodium* is psychologically insecure, lacking confidence and often feeling fearful within. To compensate for these inadequate feelings, he may strive hard in business and overwork, and he develops a "need for power." As a consequence, his emotional life suffers, he becomes hardened, has difficulty in maintaining relationships, and in general does not take responsibility in love. He becomes less trustful and fears that others will usurp his position of power. His authoritarianism is characterized by an inability to give of himself. He becomes forceful and aggressive to cover up for his insecurities, and he resorts to infantile methods of self-preservation and overprotectiveness, which are first-chakra characteristics. This problem in not giving emotionally is also reflected on the physical level and manifests as the retention and inability to give up his stool, resulting in constipation.

Pulsatilla (wind flower) is a remedy which characterizes the person with chronic diarrhea. This person is highly emotional, changeable, and suggestible. Generally, a remedy which corresponds to women, or to men who are unafraid of showing their more feminine side, *Pulsatilla* is suitable for people who do not have a strong sense of identity and are easily molded by their environment. All fluids from the body flow easily, including tears when sad or happy, nasal discharge during colds or allergies, and stools. The *Pulsatilla* personality is characterized by always wanting to give and please others. This is very similar to the diarrhea personality in the psychosomatic model.

Treatment: Mental Level

Meditation and/or psychotherapy are of paramount importance in holistic medical therapeutics in helping prevent or heal lower bowel disorders and ulcers. These practices not only treat the organic dysfunction but also enable the suffering individual to learn to understand concomitant psychological disturbances that underlie bowel and gastric problems. By becoming aware of emotional conflicts that are associated with the physical conditions of diarrhea or constipation, a person can actually transform his discomfort into a learning experience. He may observe that when he feels particularly selfish or obsessive, his bowel movements become irregular. Extreme acquisitiveness or paranoia may be noticed as leading to constipation, while extreme anxiety or apprehension may result in diarrhea or ulcer formation. Awareness is the first step in problem resolution. This is followed by taking steps to integrate the knowledge gained through self-awareness into practical methods to eliminate the digestive problems. Perhaps the person learns by careful scrutiny that wheat or milk or raw foods cause diarrhea and he then avoids them. He may discover that his breathing may be primarily from the chest, freezing the diaphragm and abdominal muscles, which leads to bowel inactivity and constipation.

Enhanced awareness of how physical habits, personality traits, and emotional conflicts lead to disorders of the digestive system can result from both psychotherapy and meditation. Through slow, methodic psychological insight, energy is redirected from creating abnormal physiologic conditions like ulcers and lower bowel disorders and is liberated to help better integrate body, mind, and spirit.

A Treatment Plan

In the case of L. W., the colitis patient discussed at the beginning of this chapter, the approach to therapy included a dietary program involving the elimination of coffee, red meat, and refined carbohydrates. Fish, poultry, and tofu (soybean curd) were recommended as high quality and non-irritating protein sources. In addition, fresh vegetables were to be cooked and fruit peeled to provide a healthy source of nonirritating roughage.

The patient began a program of regular exercise which consisted of swimming four times per week. This was chosen because she liked the sport and a public pool was available in her neighborhood.

She was also taught to practice diaphragmatic breathing and relaxation to help balance the overactivity of her parasympathetic nervous system. This also served to provide a tool for discharging the anxiety she felt with the pressures of her job.

As a result of these changes, the patient's colitis improved approximately fifty percent. Once this plateau was reached, she was given the homeopathic remedy *Lycopodium*, prescribed because it closely correponds to her symptoms of constipation alternating with diarrhea, cramping, and flatulence. Also, *Lycopodium* is helpful in diseases where lack of self-confidence is a prominent characteristic. The patient had additional symptoms of always feeling cold and strong craving for sweets, which are further indications for use of *Lycopodium*. By the fourth week after taking the remedy, the patient's colitis symptoms were completely resolved and her anxiety was much reduced, allowing her to healthfully continue her work.

16

Skin Eruptions and Acne

Miss T. is a twenty-eight-year-old woman with a history of
several skin disorders, including cystic acne since adolescence and chronic re-occurring eczema since childhood.
Both dermatologic problems got worse during times of high
emotional stress. Arguments with her mother particularly
aggravated her symptoms. Instead of expressing her opin-
ions, she either sulked or exploded in rage. In either case,
she was ill-at-ease expressing angry feelings. As a consequence, inner frustration and built-up anger manifested in
an outbreak of eczema, which she scratched until the skin
bled, as though she were attacking herself.

Her mother gave her subtle messages that she was incompetent to make her own decisions, and she slowly
developed feelings of inadequacy and in general lacked self-
confidence. Her eczema, in a sense disfiguring, reconfirmed
her negative self-image. To compound the problem, her
father constantly offered her money for vacations and lux-
uries. Despite earning a good salary, she felt obliged to
accept these monetary gifts so that her father would not be
upset. This made her feel even more dependent, which
further decreased her feelings of self-worth and self-esteem
and worsened her acne condition.

After considering the many facets of skin disorders and exploring treatments on many levels, we will present a treatment plan for this patient in the context of holistic medical practices.

Skin Physiology and Function

The skin is the largest organ in the body, weighing over eight pounds in the average male, with an area close to eighteen square feet. In the embryo, the skin is derived from a primitive type cell, the *ectoderm*, which makes up the layer of cells that surrounds the developing embryo. As the embryo grows, most of these cells remain on the outer surface and later develop into the skin. However, a small group of these cells migrate inward towards the center of the embryo, forming a structure called the neural tube. The neural tube eventually develops into the spinal cord, brain, and other nervous tissue.

Since both skin and nervous tissue originate from the same cell type, there is a close interrelationship between these two organ systems. This intimate connection is demonstrated in the ways in which the skin reflects the emotions or mental states. Blushing with embarrassment, turning white with fear, and being purple with rage are all examples of this. Many classic dermatological diseases, such as eczema, psoriasis, acne, and neurodermatitis, are associated with an underlying imbalanced emotional state.

The Skin and Protection

The skin as an organ system performs many essential functions. Primarily, it acts as a barrier to protect the internal environment from the challenges of the external world.

Skin is made up of two distinct layers. The deep layer is called the dermis, which is the origin of the nerves, blood vessels, and glandular structures like the sweat and oil glands. The more external layer is called the epidermis and contains the cells which make up what is commonly thought of as skin. As the cells at the deepest level of the epidermis divide, the older cells are pushed toward the surface where they eventually die, lose their individual shape, and merge into a single layer of essentially dead tissue. This dead tissue is primarily composed of a protein material called keratin. It is this upper layer of dead cells which gives the skin its tough consistency and provides protection against physical trauma and bacterial invasion.

Located within the skin are special cells called melanocytes. These cells function to produce a darkly colored chemical called melanin. Skin coloring is dependent upon the amount of melanin produced and the number of melanocytes in the skin: the greater their number or activity, the darker the skin. Scandinavians have relatively few melanocytes in their skin as compared to Blacks. When exposed to solar irradiation, melanocytes make more melanin to block the irradiation from passing through to the deeper levels of the skin. This serves two functions. First, it protects the skin from burning, and secondly it protects the body from overproducing Vitamin D.

The production of Vitamin D begins in the deeper layers of the skin. A reaction between the ultraviolet radiation from the sun and a fatty substance found in the skin produces the compound which ultimately becomes Vitamin D. The body needs only a limited amount of Vitamin D everyday. Overproduction of this vitamin can lead to excessive calcium absorption and possibly kidney stones. Only a small area of skin needs to be exposed to the sun to produce an adequate amount of Vitamin D. In fact, it has been estimated that a fair-skinned individual living in the tropic would only need to expose a postage-stamp-size area of skin to the sun one hour a day to produce a sufficient amount of Vitamin D. Without the protection provided by melanin, individuals living in the tropics would be in constant danger of overproducing Vitamin D and would suffer from Vitamin D toxicity.

In northern latitudes, where the sun's intensity is diminished and the weather is cold, people tend to expose less of their bodies to the sun. In the winter the days are short; hence Vitamin D production diminishes. Since Vitamin D is essential for calcium absorption and bone formation, too little Vitamin D can be just as dangerous as too much, leading to deficient calcium absorption and diseases such as rickets. As expected, rickets is more common in urban Blacks than in other groups. This is because their dark pigmentation, along with the other factors listed above, plus air pollution which blocks the sun's intensity, all predispose them to decreased Vitamin D production. Therefore, dark-skinned people living in northern urban conditions should be careful to obtain an adequate amount of Vitamin D in their diet.

Another function of the skin is to help maintain fluid and mineral balance. Through the process of sweating, the skin plays a role in regulating body temperature, water balance, and salt balance. In this sense, the skin functions as a third kidney. The skin acts as a barrier to the evaporation of water which comprises 80 percent of the body's weight. If the skin is injured, as in the case of a burn, the mechanism breaks down and large quantities of fluid and salt may exude through the skin. In serious burns the danger of dehydration resulting from fluid losses through the skin is the most immediate cause of fatality.

The Skin and Elimination

Since the skin functions as a surrogate kidney, it also has an important role to play in the elimination of wastes or toxic materials. For example, during fasting it is common for perspiration to become much more odoriferous, indicating the elimination of certain waste materials via the skin. One of the telltale symptoms of kidney failure is the appearance of a whitish discharge on the skin. Urea, a waste product produced by the body as it utilizes protein, is normally eliminated via the kidneys, but when the kidneys fail, the skin tries to compensate and urea is eliminated through perspiration producing the white discharge called uremic frost.

The importance of the skin as an eliminative organ is emphasized even more in Eastern and other holistic medical systems than in Western medicine. Skin eruptions are felt to represent the mind-body's way of throwing off processes that originate in the deeper levels of a person's psyche. If an individual is to be truly cured from a disease process, the process needs to work itself outward to the surface. Merely treating a skin eruption such as eczema with cortisone cream does not remove the underlying cause or cure the inner disease process. We have seen that this principle, that cure takes place from the inside out, is central to many holistic traditions. If a patient is treated by a homeopathic physician, for example, and comes back the next week with the complaint, "Well, since my last visit I feel much better mentally but I have this rash," the homeopath knows that the patient is getting better because the process is moving outward from the mental to the physical level.

The homeopath also views the commonly ignored eruptions on the skin such as moles and warts as being very significant. According to homeopathy, warts are the external manifestation of an internal imbalance. There is a weakness that allows this virus to grow; when the weakness is corrected, the virus will be eliminated.

The Skin: Communication and Expression

Besides functioning as an instrument of protection and excretion, the skin also serves as an organ of reception and communication. The skin contains hundreds of millions of tiny nerve endings which are sensitive to touch, pressure, and temperature, and these are important aspects of the skin's ability to perceive. These nerve endings send impulses to the brain where integration of these sensory stimuli is interpreted as pain, pleasure, pressure, heat, or cold.

More important, at least from a psychological perspective, is that the skin allows people to communicate feelings. Physical contact allows a person to "get a feeling" for another individual. A strong, firm handshake transmits a different message from a weak one, and a cold, clammy hand means something still different. A warm embrace conveys quite a different message from a casual hug. Much more can be discerned in a kiss than in the conversation that precedes it. In language, the receptive function of the skin is often used to describe perceptions, for example, "you feel so distant."

The sense of touch is the first to reach maturity in the developing infant. It has been observed that the newborn receives most of its stimulation and communication from the outside world through the skin. It takes several weeks for the eyes and ears to fully develop, but the skin is already a mature sensory organ at birth. For the newborn, the emotions associated with pleasure are fulfilled simply by the security of the mother's embrace. The skin, especially in the fetus and the newborn child, is the principle mode of communication.

Bonding between mother and child is extremely important. Many of the psychoneurotic afflictions which are common in Western society may be a result of inadequate, unsatisfactory, or negative sensory stimulation during infancy. Specific modern practices are implicated, such as early maternal-infant separation which occurs in most nurseries, the practice of bottle feeding, as well as general cultural habits such as isolating the child in a crib or carriage as opposed to carrying the infant on one's back.[1]

The expressive quality of touch is just as important as the

---

[1]Montagu, *Touching*.

specific message perceived through touch. It is as emotionally fulfilling for the mother as she gives to her child through touch as it for the baby to receive.

The Skin as a Reflection of General Health

A person's health can be ascertained by observing certain features of the skin. It is easy to distinguish a person in glowing health from a terminal patient with sunken features. In fact, studying the skin has always served as an important aspect in the art of medical diagnosis. Vitamin B deficiency may manifest as a rash or cracked lips. Zinc deficiency appears as white spots on the nails. Protein deficiency also affects the consistency of the nails, causing horizontal ridging to occur. Diabetes, cancer, gout, and most systemic illnesses have demonstrated skin symptoms.

The study of relating surface skin anatomy of the body to internal organ functions is called physiognamy. In Western medicine it is recognized that a crease on the earlobe may indicate active or latent heart disease. Coarse facial features are seen in acromegaly (excessive growth-hormone effects) and the round moon-shaped face is seen in Cushing's disease (adrenal hyperfunctioning). In traditional medical systems such as Oriental medicine, the study of facial features is highly developed, and the external is considered to be a reflection of the internal. The lines of the face, the shape of the nose and lips, and the slant of the eyes are all significant. By observing these characteristics, it becomes possible to diagnose liver, kidney, and heart problems.

Chinese Physiognomy

This phenomenon of the external reflecting the internal is most clearly established in the specific acupuncture discipline known as auriculotherapy. *Auriculo* means ear; *acupuncture* describes a point-for-point reflection of every body part on the external ear. Inserting an acupuncture needle in the point on the ear that corresponds to a particular body part will cause numbness in that body part. This is one of the major manipulations used in acupuncture anaesthesia. Similarly, in foot reflexology, the organs of the body are considered to correspond to certain areas on the soles of the feet. Pressure on a certain part of the sole may affect the corresponding body part. These two therapies represent specific parts of the body's surface on which the entire anatomy of the body is mapped out in detail.

This mirroring of the inner body upon the surface, along with other functions of the skin which have been discussed, such as elimination, protection and communication on emotional and intellectual levels, helps to explain how body massage can influence the person positively through this most sensitive receptor, the skin.

Acne and Other Eruptions

There are many types of skin eruptions, varying in color, texture, type of discharge, degree of inflammation, and intensity of pain or itching. Most eruptions, like mild acne, eczema, or seborrhea, usually represent a vent for the system's waste products. A small minority of skin problems, like certain skin cancers, severe psoriasis, or lupus erythematosis, represent deep systemic disorders which, in a sense, spill out onto the skin.

In this discussion, acne has been chosen as a prototype of a mild skin eruption because it is perhaps the most common dermatologic problem, and it is also amenable to various types of treatments. Acne therapeutics offers an interesting comparison between modern and ancient medical systems. While the major focus will be on acne, skin eruptions in general will be discussed when appropriate.

Acne is a condition of recurrent pimple formation which blocks the pores through which the sebaceous glands drain. Sebaceous gland oil backs up and seeps into the skin, creating irritation. Secondarily, bacteria may infect this area of inflammation. While most common during adolescence, acne may persist throughout adult life. Several etiologic factors have been incriminated—nutritional deficiencies or excesses, hormonal dysfunctions, psychological conflicts, and infections—but no single agent has been demonstrated to be the definitive cause of acne. Stress is important because it affects the immune system and hormone secretions. The male hormones, androgens, are known to cause acne if their levels are too high. According to Eastern and other schools of natural medicine, acne represents the body's way of expelling waste, and like other chronic diseases, is a manifestation of an underlying imbalance.

Treatment: Physical Level

Cleanliness is an important preventive in the treatment of acne. Washing helps to reduce surface dirt and oil which may clog skin pores, thus allowing the secretion of the sebaceous gland (sebum) to drain normally. The sebum has antibacterial and antifungal properties and protects and lubricates the skin.

When cleansing is not sufficient to prevent acne, standard treatment in Western medicine usually consists of antibiotic creams and pills to destroy the bacteria growing on the face, which add to the inflammation by producing secondary infection. Initially this approach seems beneficial, yet its effects are only temporary. The skin improves only so long as the antibiotics are continued. As soon as they are stopped, the acne flares up, often more severely than before. Another factor not often associated with the use of antibiotics, is the effect these drugs can have on the intricate relationship between the bacteria living on the skin and the skin itself. Normal skin bacteria are destroyed by the antibiotics and they are replaced by new and often drug-resistant bacteria. Furthermore, it is not only the skin's bacteria which are affected when an antibiotic is taken, but the bacterial population of the throat, colon, or vagina may also be altered. When this occurs, the person becomes more susceptible to sore throats, various intestinal difficulties, or recurrent vaginitis.

As the bacteria on the skin become resistant to routine antibiotics, new and often more powerful antibiotics must be used. This approach is akin to using insecticides to treat disease in plants. Although initially the insecticide may appear helpful as it destroys the pest, it also has a destructive affect on those organisms that have a beneficial relationship with the plant. Eventually the whole ecosystem is altered. Resistant insects or new pests begin to appear. The yield decreases and the farmer must then try new and often more lethal chemicals, changing periodically, as one insecticide after another becomes ineffective.

From a holistic medical perspective, *nutrition* is of utmost importance in preventing acne. It is often helpful to avoid animal fats, refined carbohydrates, chocolate, and foods with preservatives. Fresh fruits, vegetables, whole grains, legumes, and lean meats should be emphasized. Zinc and Vitamins A, B complex, and C have a therapeutic effect on acne. Because of its high Vitamin A content, carrot juice is helpful.

Performing yoga washes such as the upper wash has been advocated, the rationale being that these washes help the body eliminate waste products and mucus that would otherwise be discharged through the skin and mucus membranes. (See Appendix.) Sun exposure, clay, salt packs, and other external applications often prove useful. Steaming the face is also recommended. For people with oily skin, the following process can help dry up the face, clean out blackheads, and close off pores. Bring water to a boil, then add rosemary leaves and continue boiling for sixty seconds longer. Turn off the heat and place a towel over the head and pot so that the vapor with the rosemary essence gently envelopes the face. Keep the face far enough away from the pot so as not to scald it with the rising steam. Continue for approximately five minutes. Then wash the face with a gentle abrasive soap, such as almond or oatmeal, and warm water. A louffa sponge can also be used to brush off dead scales. A cool-water rinse should follow to close the opened pores.

Vigorous *active exercise* is often helpful in acne and other types of skin eruptions as increased blood circulation to the skin stimulates stagnant areas where sebum and bacteria build up. The induction of perspiration may also help eliminate metabolic and stored environmental waste products. Some people never sweat, and when this function is re-established they find their general health improves because perspiration serves as a natural vent for accumulated waste material. Thus, sauna baths and steam baths are also advantageous therapy for acne.

Hatha yoga has a positive effect on skin problems because, through the performance of postures, relaxation is enhanced, hormone levels are balanced, and an increased awareness of breathing and psychological difficulties is established. Inverted postures are especially helpful because of the shunting of blood to the face and head and the subsequent cleansing effect.

Treatment: Energy and Mental Levels

Breathing. The practice of diaphragmatic breathing and relaxation is essential in the treatment of acne. Stress, psychological conflicts, and resultant hormonal imbalances are important in the etiology of acne. Diaphragmatic breathing and relaxation help to direct emotional responses toward more stable and creative directions. This simple practice can markedly affect the influence of stress upon the autonomic nervous system and the endocrine (hormone) system.

Other breathing exercises are very beneficial in skin disorders, especially if a slow and gradual increase in capacity is established. Kapalabhati, if vigorously practiced, can exert a cleansing effect on the skin as a fine perspiration is released. (See Appendix.) Gently rubbing this perspiration is said by advanced practitioners to add a healthy glow to the complexion.

Homeopathy. The human body is a highly resilient and adaptable structure and, if not severely tested, will maintain homeostasis. But if it is continuously overwhelmed by a combination of stresses like poor quality nutrition, lack of exercise, and emotional strain, the body's ability to maintain normal physiologic functioning may break down. In this situation, the skin, representing the most external and superficial of the body's organs, can be the area onto which all inner processes are reflected.

Holistic medicine maintains that physical health is dependent on optimal functioning of the eliminative systems, including the urinary, respiratory, and digestive tracts. The liver is also intricately involved in cleansing processes, as it promotes the degradation and metabolism of toxins, drugs, and chemicals. If any of these vital body parts is dysfunctional, the skin becomes an alternative organ of elimination and begins to discharge these waste products. From this perspective, skin eruptions such as acne or eczema are really a systemic problem representing inner disorder.

Emotional health also has manifestations on the skin. Because the skin and nervous system are closely related, the skin will reflect imbalances of the nervous system.

Homeopathic medicine asserts that the depth and degree of illness depends on: (1) inherited predisposition; (2) the intensity of a stressful stimulus, whether environmental, accidental, emotional, or micro-organism overgrowth; and (3) the nature of the treatment used in terms of strengthening or weakening the defense mechanism.

When the mind and/or body are disturbed, the natural reaction of the human organism is to attempt to re-establish order and homeostasis. Since the vital force will protect the most vital structures by creating a zone of defense at the most superficial and least harmful levels, symptoms will manifest as far from the more important organs as possible. Thus the skin, being the most superficial area, has the most symptoms manifest upon it. From this perspective, skin eruptions are reflections of a defense reaction and are actually protective in nature.

Homeopaths consider it to be a dangerous and poor prognostic sign if the patient displays signs of illness yet does not have the vitality and inner power to throw off the disordered processes onto the skin in the form of heat (fever), rashes, pimples, boils, or eczema. In this situation, the internal organs, or even the mind, stay afflicted with the disease process. Another unfavorable situation can arise when drugs are continuously used to suppress skin manifestations. When this superficial point of defense is removed, a new more internal barrier must be created. Because the original attempt of the system to establish balance was the best possible at that particular moment, the new level occurring after suppression would probably be worse. Thus, if every time psoriasis, eczema, or abscesses erupt, their outlets are obstructed by drugs like cortisone or coal tar preparations, then the defense mechanism, which was attempting to establish homeostasis by eliminating the disease process on the most peripheral level possible (skin), is inhibited and the vital force is weakened. A secondary defense is established at a less superficial level, which is less effective, more internal, and consequently more threatening to the organism. A shock or external stimulus, which would normally be neutralized by a strong vital force acting through the defense mechanism, may now overwhelm the weakened vital force. It is in this sense that the disease process is said to have been driven inward to more vital areas.

Silicea or pure flint is a homeopathic remedy whose mode of action exemplifies the idea that the system attempts to reestablish homeostasis by expulsion through the skin. The close connection between emotions and personality characteristics and the skin's physical symptomatology also becomes apparent through analysis of this homeopathically prepared mineral. *Silicea* helps to localize and open abcesses since it promotes suppuration (pus formation). It seems to stimulate a weakened vital force to throw out infectious processes or hardened tissues, as well as foreign bodies like splinters. In a constitution that seems to lack the necessary strength to establish a strong defense at its periphery (skin), *Silicea* gives the vital force an extra push to complete the process. Boils or pimples are stimulated to come to a head, and they begin to drain; scar tissue is absorbed and subsequently softens; and old cracks or fistulous openings on the skin heal.

It is interesting to note that the microscopic nature of flint is characterized by very tiny yet extremely sharp points. The essence of *Silicea* reflects this configuration in that its sharp edge seems to "cut open" the skin so that the disease process can find a vent.

Physical feebleness and lack of reactivity is closely associated with a concomitant mental weakness. A person who requires *Silicea* is typically "yielding, faint-hearted, anxious, sensitive to all impressions, has a lack of vital heat, is cold and chilly, and in general has a want of grit, moral or physical."[2] Another quote from one of the most brilliant homeopaths of the late nineteenth and early twentieth centuries, James Tyler Kent, M. D., eloquently exemplifies the peculiar mental state of the typical patient that responds to *Silicea:*

> The patient lacks stamina. What *Silicea* is to the stalk of grain in the field, it is to the human mind. Take the glossy, stiff, outer covering of a stalk of grain and examine it, and you will realize with what firmness it supports the head of grain until it ripens; there is a gradual deposit of *Silicea* in it to give it stamina. So it is with the mind; when the mind needs *Silicea* it is in a state of weakness, embarrassment, dread, a state of yielding. If you should listen to the description of this state by a prominent clergyman or a lawyer, or a man in the habit of appearing in public with self-confidence, firmness and fullness of thought and speech, he would tell you he had come to a state where he dreads to appear in public, he feels his own selfhood so

---

[2]W. Boericke, *Material Medica with Reperatory.* New Delhi: Jain Publishing Co., 1976, p. 891.

that he cannot enter into his subject, he dreads it, he fears that he will fail, his mind will not work, he is worn out by prolonged efforts at mental work. But he will say that when he forces himself into the harness he can go on with ease, his usual self-command returns to him and he does well; he does his work with promptness, fullness and accuracy. The peculiar *Silicea* state is found in the dread of failure. If he has any unusual mental task to perform, he fears he will make a failure of it, yet he does it well. This is the early state; of course there comes a time when he cannot perform the work with accuracy and he may need *Silicea*.[3]

The homeopathic remedy *Sulphur* offers another interesting study of mind-body-skin interrelatedness. Mentally, a person needing *Sulphur* is irritable, volatile, angry, and emotionally eruptive. He tends to argue vehemently about all sorts of meaningless issues and is called "the ragged philosopher." As J. T. Kent says:

He has long, uncut hair and a dirty face; his study is uncleanly, it is untidy; books and leaves of books are piled up indiscriminately; there is no order. It seems that *Sulphur* produces this state of disorder, a state of untidiness, a state of uncleanliness, a state of "I don't care how things go," and a state of selfishness. He becomes a false philosopher, and the more he goes on in this state the more he is disappointed because the world does not consider him the greatest man on earth.[4]

The *Sulphur* skin is characterized by a similar eruptive nature. All sorts of eruptions occur; vesicular, pustular, scaly, herpetic, eczematous. Like its corresponding hot-tempered personality, the *Sulphur* discharges are hot, corrosive, and burning. As the *Sulphur* patient is unclean and odoriferous generally, the discharges are also foul-smelling.

[3]Kent, *Lectures on Homeopathic Materia Medica*, p. 925-926.
[4]Ibid, p. 952.

Another prominent skin symptom of the *Sulphur* type illness is that intense itching accompanies most problems. This is particularly aggravated by wool, warm rooms or beds, and baths (the *Sulphur* patient despises bathing), and is generally worse at night. Relief often is afforded through voluptuous scratching until the skin becomes raw and begins to burn.

Psychosomatic medicine describes severe scratching as an expression of hostile, angry impulses that have been deflected from their real target and turned against oneself. Often, the reason such a person does not express his anger or hostility is because he feels guilty about them. Often parents or society mistakenly convey to children that it is not right to feel or express hostile or angry feelings. Sexual repression can also lead to held-in guilt or frustration, which can result in pent-up anger. Scratching serves as an outlet for these repressed hostile feelings, and as the person scratches furiously to cause scabbing and bleeding, the resulting disfigurement can lead to shame and humiliation which may cause others to reject him. This helps to promote an attitude—that "I am no good anyway," which can serve to ease the feelings of underlying guilt.

The *Sulphur* patient seems to react in a similar fashion to that presented by the psychosomatic scheme. The *Sulphur* anger and hostility are either expressed in volatile outbursts or are repressed and sublimated into other areas like study or philosophical dissertation. This work, however, is disorderly and disorganized as the misdirected and dissipated focus of attention makes the quality of the work poor. The repressed anger is also expressed as uncleanliness or extreme scratching that eventually causes the skin to become raw, red, and ugly. Both situations become a mechanism to keep other people away or to cause rejection by others. Thus the guilt that arose from hostile impulses is expiated.

From the above discussion, it should be clear that acne is dependent on a variety of factors. It is not due solely to the facial bacteria, too much chocolate or pizza, or hormonal problems. Acne can flourish only when the right bacteria begin to grow in a receptive environment prepared by faulty nutrition, an unhealthy psychological matrix, and disruptive physiological changes associated with adolescence or the menstrual cycle.

The skin is a mirror of health; the color, glow, dryness, or oiliness of the skin are reflections of a person's internal condition. Organ dysfunctions manifest themselves on the skin. Likewise, unresolved emotional issues often appear as skin problems. Therefore, a healthy skin often reflects a healthy personality. The approach to an unhealthy skin is not to apply creams but to work on correcting the internal imbalance through following a good nutritional program and through trying to identify and confront psychological problems.

A Treatment Plan

Treatment for Miss T., the patient presented at the beginning of the chapter, was multifaceted. Nutritionally, she was taken off all animal fats including beef, pork, and eggs. Lighter vegetable oils such as cold pressed sesame, sunflower seed, and olive oils were allowed. Dairy products were restricted, not only because the fat seemed to make her acne worse, but also because she proved to be allergic to the milk protein, which exacerbated her eczema. Specific supplements that were helpful included for the acne Vitamins A and C and Zinc, as well as the herbs Golden Seal and Echinacea. For the eczema Vitamin B was added. She was advised to keep areas of eczema dry and exposed to sunlight, and a combination of oil of Calendula (Marigold), Vitamin E, and sesame oil was used topically. A facial sauna and herbal clay packs were prescribed for her facial acne. The cleansing breathing techniques, Kapalabhati and Bhramari, were practiced daily. (See Appendix.) Several homeopathic remedies were used, the most important being *Graphites* (Graphite) when her eczema oozed a sticky substance and she was depressed and constipated, *Sepia* (ink of the female cuttlefish) when she was withdrawn and her acne and eczema erupted premenstrually, and *Sulphur* when her anger was self-directed and she scratched her eczema until it bled.

Relaxation techniques and diaphragmatic breathing helped her realize how tight her muscles were. She quickly learned good control over skin temperature changes by using biofeedback. Slowly through psychotherapy, she began to recognize her anger and learned to confront her parents more directly when they discouraged her efforts to assert herself. She began to refuse her father's money and moved into her own apartment. She generally assumed a more honest and mature relationship with her parents. Simultaneously, the intensity of her eczema reactions diminished and her acne greatly improved.

Epilogue

By now the reader will have noted that there are several dimensions to holism as it applies to healing. First, as has been emphasized again and again, holism means a perspective where body, mind, and spirit are of equal importance in maintenance of health and in treatment of disease. We have presented a model from yoga philosophy which allows all levels of consciousness to be brought into perspective for each individual case.

In addition, holism is the area of medicine based on ancient tenets, more recent changes in orthodox medicine, and on future ideals. The integration of technology with the psychospiritual dimensions of man underlies this approach. In the integrated model we have presented, ancient and modern systems can complement one another in a cohesive and universal manner. We have tried to show specifically how ancient methodologies and concepts can be used to reach a fuller and more complete understanding of an illness, and we have provided cases and sample treatment plans to indicate ways to reach all the levels of the disease process. We do not mean to imply that the systems of medicine presented here are the only or the best, but we have discussed only those therapies and approaches that we have thoroughly tested through our own medical practice. Our aim has been practical, to furnish both concepts by which to understand health and disease and methods of treatment.

There is a third dimension to holistic medicine which we have touched upon but not spelled out fully. This involves the responsibilities of the holistic physician and also those of the patient, and it indicates the most effective kind of relationship between them.

For a holistic physician to practice quality medicine in the most consistent, intelligent, and ethical manner, it is essential that he assume certain responsibilities. (1) He must keep up with modern advances, both in orthodox medicine and in new findings concerning the ancient methods and theories. (2) He must refer patients to appropriate specialists when necessary. (3) He must become thoroughly familiar with alternative methods of healing when they have become well proven. (4) He must individualize treatment. (5) Part of the ideal of holistic treatment is to keep costs down. (6) The patient must be taught self-care techniques and learn to improve his own health, becoming less dependent on the physician. (7) Through explaining both theory and treatment to the patient, the physician should demystify medical care. (8) This involves open communication with the patient on many issues. (9) The physician must become a role model, inspiring patients to live holistically. This means that he must himself practice approaches inherent in holism, being both a healer and personally a practitioner of health.

Of equal importance is the patient's responsibility of being compliant and receptive without being passive. Norman Cousins described the ideal patient as one who: "(1) does not require a prescription to demonstrate he is getting his money's worth, (2) does not believe that the best medications are necessarily represented by the latest and most powerful chemical concoctions, (3) does not feel insulted if he is told by the doctor that his problem is psychogenic and not organic, (4) does not dump his symptoms on the doctor's table and expect the full responsibility for cure, and (5) does not panic at the first sign of pain."[1] The patient must take responsibility for his own health and become involved in his treatment.

We would like to add two more responsibilities to the list that apply both to the holistic physician and the holistic patient. To really work, patient and doctor must have mutual trust in one another. In addition, they must share two mutual goals. First, they must both believe in the idea of self-healing, and second, they must have the conviction that a person can grow and learn from illness as well as from health. They must look at pain and suffering as leading to greater awareness and compassion, as catalysts to both insight and action—all of which leads to physical, emotional, and spiritual freedom. Thus "getting well" is only the beginning of a life-long journey toward wholeness and health at all levels, spirit, mind, and body.

In writing this book, we wanted to share our approaches with others in an attempt to offer guidance to those looking for a more humanistic way to understand psyche and soma. We wanted to show how ancient approaches and modern systems are in many ways similar, thus bridging the gap between the past, present, and future. We wanted to inspire people to learn to care for themselves and to live life with vigor and strength of mind and body. But most of all, we wanted to share the excitement and insight that we have gained through our professional and personal journey into the marvels and mysteries of being human. We humbly hope we have served our purposes.

---

[1]C. Lough and B. Stewart, *Self Care as a Health Service* (Chapter 8), in R. F. Rushmer, ed., *National Priorities for Health: Past, Present, and Projected.* New York: John Wiley and Sons, 1980, p. 307.

Practical Techniques of Holistic Medicine

Breathing Exercises

Complete Yoga Breath

Technique
1. Sit with your head, neck, and trunk in a straight line. Breathe smoothly and gently.
2. Inhale slowly and deeply, allowing the abdomen to protrude to the furthest extent. There should be no strain.
3. Without pause, begin to fill the chest cavity so that it flares out to its maximum, again without undue strain. The abdomen may contract inwards slightly as the chest expands.
4. Without pause, raise the clavicles (collar bones) slightly.
5. After reaching the maximum inhalation, do not pause but begin to exhale, following the opposite sequence as inhalation.
6. On exhalation, the clavicles should be allowed to lower slightly.
7. Without pause, the chest cavity should relax inwards.
8. Without pause, contract the abdominal muscles inwards to their maximum, again without strain.
9. After completing the fullest and deepest exhalation, this exercise may be repeated 2-8 times.
10. This exercise should not be repeated too often because it can lead to over-stimulation.

Physical Benefits
1. Aerates the entire lungs.
2. Decreases the amount of dead space in the lungs and in the residual capacity.

3. Exercises and strengthens respiratory muscles.
4. Stimulates sympathetic nervous system.
5. Stimulates stretch receptors of lungs.
6. Increases oxygen to tissues in the brain.
7. Decreases diseases such as asthma, bronchitis, and pneumonia.
8. Flushes out conducting system.
9. Stimulates digestive system.
10. Stimulates the heart.

Psychospiritual Benefits
1. Brings greater awareness to the respiratory phases.
2. Helps emotional problems related to restricted diaphragm.
3. Re-energizes by bringing increased prana to the nadis.
4. Helps bring greater control to the fourth chakra.

Alternate Nostril Breathing

Technique
1. Always sit with your head, neck, and trunk straight, facing front, and let the breath be relaxed and even.
2. There are three variations to alternate nostril breathing. Any of these is acceptable if it is consistently practiced (don't change to other variations). Using your right hand, block off the left nostril with your your 4th and 5th fingers and block off the right nostril with your thumb.
   A. Exhale through the active (more open) nostril and inhale through the passive (more closed) nostril three times. After a third inhalation through the passive nostril, reverse the process and exhale through the passive and inhale through the active nostril three times. Drop hands to knees and do three complete inhalations and exhalations. This completes one cycle. Do one to three cycles.

Exhale	*Inhale*
Active	Passive
Active	Passive
Active	Passive
Passive	Active
Passive	Active
Passive	Active

B. Exhale through the passive side and inhale through the passsive side three times. Then exhale through the active side and inhale through the active side three times. Do three complete inhalations and exhalations. This completes one cycle. Do one to three cycles.

Exhale	Inhale
Passive	Passive
Passive	Passive
Passive	Passive
Active	Active
Active	Active
Active	Active

C. Exhale and inhale through the passive side, then exhale and inhale through the active side. Exhale and inhale through the passive side. Continue alternating each side, exhaling out and inhaling back through the same side. On the third exhalation and inhalation through the active side, exhale and inhale through both nostrils three times. This is one cycle. Do one to three cycles.

Exhale	Inhale
Passive	Passive
Active	Active
Passive	Passive
Active	Active
Passive	Passive
Active	Active

Physical Benefits
1. Improves sense of smell.
2. Removes excess mucus from nose.
3. Shrinks membranes to help relieve nasal congestion.
4. Prevents upper respiratory infections.
5. Enhances digestion by being able to keep right nostril open.
6. Balances parasympathetic and sympathetic functioning, creating physiological equilibrium.

Psychospiritual Benefits
1. Promotes relaxation and calmness.
2. Promotes meditative moods (often exercise is done before meditation).

3. Balances nadis.
4. Helps avert emotional storms.
5. Helps observation of subtle pranic (energy) flow and gradually helps to mentally alter the flow.

Breath Awareness

Technique

1. Watching the breath flow can be done in all situations, such as walking, reading, listening to discussions, or driving. Stressful conditions are especially appropriate for breath awareness. Before and during meditation are times when breath awareness is essential.
2. There are several different methods for observing the breath flow.
   A. Mentally observe the abdominal wall rising upwards while inspiring and falling while expiring.
   B. Mentally observe the breath flow through the nose. During inspiration, trace the coolness up to the root of the nose, and then feel the warmth of the breath as it passes out during exhalation.
3. Practice breath awareness for any length of time and as often as desired.
4. Be sure to eliminate any noise, jerks, or pauses. The breath should flow only through the nose.
5. The breathing should be diaphragmatic, with the chest remaining relatively stationary.
6. The breath should be slow, smooth, and relatively deep.
7. Inhalation and exhalation should be approximately the same length in duration (or exhalation can be drawn out a little longer).

Physical Benefits
1. Decreases sympathetic activity.
2. Creates a balance between parasympathetic and sympathetic activity.

Psychospiritual Benefits
1. Minimizes stress and tension.
2. Useful as a concentration or meditative device.
3. Useful as a precursor to meditation. Helps a person learn

to objectively observe thought patterns and emotions that are dissipating. Also helps to channel those positive thoughts and emotions into creative endeavors.

4. Helps in observing pranic currents, and helps change disruptive energy flow.

Bhramari

Technique

1. Sit with your head, neck, and trunk in a straight line. Breathe gently and smoothly.
2. Exhale completely using only the abdominal muscles which contract inwards. At the same time contract the palate and throat areas to make a low-pitched noise that sounds like the buzz of a bee.
3. Without pausing, inhale with the abdominal muscles expanding outwards. The chest cavity remains stationary. Again contracting the palate and throat areas make a high-pitched noise that resembles the buzz of a bee.
4. More resistance will be felt during inhalation. Therefore it will be more difficult to make a smooth, clear, melodious bee-like sound during inhalation than during exhalation.
5. Repeat Bhramari from one to three minutes.

Physical Benefits

1. Helps remove excess mucus and phlegm from upper respiratory passages.
2. Helps prevent or palliate tonsillitis and pharyngitis.
3. Stimulates sinuses and helps drainage from sinuses.
4. Helps stimulate and balance thyroid abnormalities.
5. Stimulates eustachian tubes and thus promotes drainage from middle ear. This helps prevent or palliate inner ear infections.
6. Palliates or prevents laryngitis.
7. Improves quality and tone of the singing and speaking voice.

Psychospiritual Benefits

1. Helps bring greater relaxation and awareness to the fifth center of consciousness (chakra).
2. Enhances ability to communicate by decreasing tension in voice box area.

3. Enhances creativity, a fifth chakra attribute.
4. Helps bring about smooth transmission of prana and udana pranas.
5. After many years of practice, induces peaceful and expanded states of consciousness.

Kapalabhati

Technique
1. Sit with your head, neck, and trunk in a straight line. Breathe gently and smoothly.
2. Forcibly and quickly exhale. Only the abdomen should move. It contracts inwards towards the back. The chest cavity remains relatively stationary.
3. Allow the inhalation to be passive, gentle, slow, and natural. The abdomen relaxes outwards with the chest again not moving.
4. The inhalation should last between two and four times as long as the exhalation.
5. Repeat between seven and twenty-one times. This makes one cycle. Repeat up to three cycles.

Physical Benefits
1. Improves oxygen exchange in lungs.
2. Promotes aeration of parts of lung normally stagnant; thus helpful in preventing build up of micro-organisms that cause pneumonia or tuberculosis.
3. Stimulates and tones bronchi and muscles surrounding bronchi, and thus is useful in preventing or palliating asthma and bronchitis.
4. Stimulates and cleanses nose, sinuses, and throat and is thus helpful in pharyngitis, rhinitis, sinusitis, laryngitis, and allergies.
5. Stimulates abdominal organs because of the strength of the diaphragmatic movement and is thus helpful in digestive problems, flatulence, liver dysfunction, and constipation.

Psychospiritual Benefits
1. Stimulates stretch reflexes of the lungs that interconnect with the parasympathetic vagus nerve; feedback with higher brain centers brings about better control of the autonomic nervous system and emotions.

2. Regulates incoming prana and outgoing apana.
3. Stimulates three chakra areas: the fourth chakra because of its proximity to the lung area; the third chakra by the strong abdominal movements; and the fifth center, which is stimulated by the breath moving quickly through the pharyngeal area.

Eye and Facial Muscle Massage

Technique
1. Rub the forehead with the fatty pad of the thumbs. Using circular motions, gradually move towards the temples. Repeat this seven times.
2. Rub the tip of the thumb across the bony area just above the eyes. Begin near the nose and move out towards the temples. Repeat seven times.
3. Rub the tip of the index finger across the bony area just below the eye. Begin near the nose and move out towards the temple. Repeat seven times.
4. Rub the tip of the index finger across the bony area next to the nose. Begin at the root of the nose (between the eyes) and move downwards past the wing of the nose. Repeat this seven times.
5. Rub the temples with the thumb's fat pad seven times.
6. Rub the muscle between the two jaws just below the ear. Repeat seven times.

Washes

Nasal Wash

Technique
1. Materials to be used: a small pot with a narrow spout, warm water, and noniodized salt. (Iodine will irritate the delicate membranes in the nose.) The water should be just salty enough so that you can taste the salt (like tears), and

the water should be comfortably warm, not hot.

2. Two variations of the nasal wash are:

A. *Side to side.* Fill the nasal wash pot. Insert the spout into the active (open) nostril. Hold your head at about a 45° angle to the ground as water goes in the active nostril and out the passive one. Reverse the sides and repeat.

B. *Nostril to Mouth.* This may be done at the same time as side to side nasal wash if the head is at the proper angle. With your head tilted sideways as in first exercise, keep your forehead raised and the throat relaxed. Close off one nostril with one hand and pour the water into the other nostril. Water will drain into the mouth. Switch nostrils and repeat.

3. Clear the water from the nose very gently. When blowing the nose, use quick forceful exhalations without closing off the nostrils with the fingers.

4. The following exercises are used for clearing water that may have accumulated in the sinuses:

A. *Opposite hand to opposite toe.* Have your head centered with your arms stretched out at shoulder height and parallel to the ground. Do not move your neck muscles. Exhale, touching your right hand to your left toes. Inhale as you return to erect posture. Repeat this three times on each side, slowly.

B. *Looking over shoulder.* Position yourself on your hands and knees with back straight. Exhale and rotate your head, looking over your shoulder. Inhale as you move back to the center. Exhale looking over the other shoulder. Inhale as you move back to center. Repeat three times on each side, slowly.

Physical Benefits

1. Drains excess mucus.
2. Heals irritated, dry, caked mucus membranes.
3. Helps drain sinuses, preventing sinusitis.
4. Helps drain eustachian tubes, preventing otitis media (ear infection).
5. Prevents, palliates, and cures upper respiratory infections and influenza.
6. Prevents, palliates, and cures sore throats and tonsillitis.
7. Enhances sense of smell.

8. Opens up clogged passageways due to deviated septum or chronic rhinitis.

Psychospiritual Benefits
1. Promotes awareness of emotions, thoughts, and instincts by stimulating nerve endings.
2. Helps balance left and right sides (see alternate nostril breathing for details).
3. Creates unobstructed vehicle for pranic flow, creating balanced energy formations.

The Upper Wash

Caution
1. The upper wash should only be done under the guidance of an experienced teacher and/or physician.
2. People with hiatal hernias, ulcers, or esophageal diseases should avoid doing the upper wash. People with hypertension or kidney disease should avoid the upper wash because of the salt content of the water.

Technique
1. Drink as rapidly as possible about 1-1/2 to 4 quarts of warm, salty water. The mixture of water to salt is about 2 teaspoons of salt per quart.
2. When you feel you can drink no more, force yourself to continue drinking until you feel that you will vomit.
3. Then place your finger in the back of the throat and regurgitate as much of the water as possible.
4. Adding the juice of half a lemon can make the water more palatable and can increase the quantity of mucus expelled.

Physical Benefits
1. Helps remove excessive mucus from the stomach.
2. The act of vomiting helps alleviate excess tension in the throat and abdominal area.
3. Useful in the treatment of asthma, especially if done in the early stages.
4. Useful in conditions of excess mucus production, such as allergies.
5. Stimulates digestion and is therefore helpful to individuals with weak digestion.

Exercise Hints

1. Exercise on a regular basis. A minimum of three to four times a week is necessary to achieve proper aerobic condition.
2. Stretching: You should spend at least five to ten minutes stretching the legs, back, and shoulders before and after exercising.
3. Pacing: In aerobics, the key is pacing; performing at a level commensurate with your ability. There is a fine line between conditioning yourself and exhausting yourself. Perhaps the easiest way to pace yourself is to exercise at a rate where you can comfortably breath through the nose, keeping the mouth closed. Other alternatives include testing the pulse and maintaining a pulse of 120, or exerting yourself at a rate at which you can easily carry on a conversation while exercising.
4. Go slowly: Most individuals when trying to get in shape are in too much of a hurry. If you have not run in many years, you cannot expect to run a five minute mile. In order to get maximum benefit from exercise, you need to spend a minimum of 20 to 30 minutes jogging or 45 minutes walking at a continuous pace. In order to do this, you need to go slowly and exercise at a comfortable pace.
5. Pain and Soreness: Anyone who exercises may experience some form of injury. Usually this is mild and self-limited such as a pulled muscle, a slight bruise, or sprain, though sometimes it can be more serious. One way to distinguish the seriousness of an injury is the exercise test. By continuing to exercise after the onset of mild pain, either the pain will disappear, indicating a mild injury, or the pain will get worse. If the latter occurs, then a period of rest is indicated, and if pain persists, then medical care should be sought. Remember, however, that a pulled muscle or sprain need not become a reason to drop out of exercising. It is normal to have some muscular soreness when starting an exercise program and this will normally diminish quickly. During the first twenty-four hours, soaking the sore areas in cool baths can be helpful to reduce pain and promote healing. After the first day warm soaks can be used.

Progressive Relaxation

Progressive relaxation is based on a technique of tightening and relaxing the various voluntary muscles in sequence to induce total body relaxation. This method is especially useful in helping individuals that are particularly tense or who have not been able to relax using breathing or mental focusing. Below is a sample progressive relaxation.

1. Lie on the back, legs 18 inches apart, arms 8-12 inches from the sides, palms up.
Bring the attention to the face. Begin tightening the facial muscles, trying to squeeze all the skin on the face toward the tip of the nose. Hold for 10 seconds and relax. Notice how this feels.
2. Next contract the muscles of the face in the opposite direction, stretching the skin away from the nose. Open the mouth, raise the eyebrows. Stretch! Hold for 10 seconds, then relax. Notice how this feels.
3. Tighten the muscles of the throat, hold 5 seconds and relax. Notice how this feels.
4. Tighten the neck muscles, pushing the head against the floor, pushing hard. Keep the other muscles relaxed. Hold 5 seconds and relax. Notice how this feels.
5. Bend the head towards the chest, as strongly as you can. Keep the shoulders and other muscles relaxed. Hold 5 seconds, then relax. Notice how this feels.
6. Tighten the shoulders, shrugging them up. While keeping the rest of the body relaxed, tighten only the shoulder muscles. Hold 5 seconds and relax. Notice how this feels.
7. Pull the shoulder muscles down toward the hips. Keep the other muscles relaxed. Hold 5 seconds and relax. Notice how this feels.
8. Push the shoulders into the floor. Push hard. Keep the rest of the body relaxed. Hold 5 seconds. Relax. Notice how this feels.
9. Tighten only the muscles of the upper arms, not the hands. Only the biceps and triceps. Hold 5 seconds and relax. Notice how this feels.
10. Tighten the forearms only, not the hands. Hold 5 seconds. Relax. Notice how this feels.
11. Tighten the hands. Make a tight fist; make it tighter, tighter. Hold 5 seconds. Relax. Notice how this feels.
12. Tighten all the muscles in the back. Push the torso against the floor. Keep the rest of the muscles relaxed. Hold 5 seconds. Relax. Notice how this feels.
13. Tighten the abdominal muscles, and only the abdominal muscles. Hold 5 seconds. Relax. Notice how this feels.
14. Squeeze the buttocks together, tight, contracting all the

muscles in the pelvis. Keep the rest of the muscles relaxed. Hold for 5-10 seconds. Relax. Notice how this feels.

15. Tighten only the thighs, keeping the rest of the body relaxed. Hold 10 seconds. Relax. Notice how this feels.
16. Tighten only the calves; hold 5 seconds. Relax. Notice how this feels.
17. Curl the toes downward tightly as possible. Hold 5 to 10 seconds. Relax. Notice how this feels.
18. Bend the toes upward, stretching the calf. Hold 5 to 10 seconds. Relax and notice how this feels.
19. Stretch the entire body from head to toe. Hold 5 to 10 seconds. Relax and notice how this feels.

Selected Bibliography

Holistic Medicine

Airola, Paavo, N.D., Ph.D. *Everywoman's Book.*
  Phoenix: Health Plus Publishers, 1979.
_____. *How to Get Well.* Phoenix: Health Plus Publishers,
  1974.
Benson, H. *The Relaxation Response.* New York: Avon,
  Morrow, 1976.
Berkeley Holistic Health Center. *The Holistic Health
  Handbook.* Berkeley: And/Or Press, 1978.
Bloomfield, H. H., and Kory, R. *The Holistic Way to
  Health and Happiness.* New York: Simon and
  Schuster, 1978.
Cousins, Norman. *Anatomy of an Illness.* New York: W.
  W. Norton, 1979.
Dubos, Rene. *Man Adapting.* New Haven: Yale University
  Press, 1980.
_____. *Man, Medicine, and Environment.* New York:
  Praeger, 1968.
_____. *Mirage of Health, Utopian Progress and Biological
  Change.* New York: Perennial Library, Harper and
  Row, 1979.
Gerras, Charles, ed., *The Encyclopedia of Common
  Diseases.* Rodale Press, Prevention Magazine, 1970.
Goldwag, Elliott, ed., *Inner Balance, The Power of
  Holistic Healing.* New York: Prentice Hall, 1979.
Jaffe, Dennis, Ph.D. *Healing from Within.* New York:
  Alfred Knopf, 1980.
Long, James, M.D. *The Essential Guide to Prescription
  Drugs.* New York: Harper and Row, 1982.

Mendelsohn, Robert, M.D. *Confessions of a Medical Heretic.* Chicago: Contemporary Books, 1979.

Muramoto, Naboru. *Healing Ourselves,* Comp. by M. Abeksera. New York: Avon, 1974.

Papenoe, Chris. *Wellness.* Washington, D.C.: Yes! Inc., 1977.

Poynter, F.N.C., ed., *Medicine and Culture.* Wellcome Institute of the History of Medicine, Frank Cottrell, LTS, 1969.

Rama, Swami. *Practical Guide to Holistic Health.* Honesdale, PA: Himalayan Institute Press, 1978.

Samuels, M., and Bennett, H. *The Well Body Book.* Westminster, MD: Random House, 1973.

Shealy, C. Norman. *Ninety Days to Self-Health.* New York: Dial/Delacourte, 1977.

_____. *The Pain Game.* Millbrae, CA: Celestial Arts, 1976.

Simonton, O.C., Matthews-Simonton, S., and Creighton, J. *Getting Well Again.* Los Angeles: J. P. Tarcher, 1978.

Sobel, David, ed., *Ways of Health: Holistic Approaches to Ancient and Contemporary Medicine.* New York: Harcourt Brace, Jovanovich, 1979.

Thomas, Lewis. *The Lives of a Cell: Notes of a Biology Watcher.* New York: Bantam, 1975.

Weil, Andrew. *Health and Healing.* Boston: Houghton Mifflin, 1983.

_____. *The Natural Mind.* Boston: Houghton Mifflin, 1972.

Chinese Medicine

Blofeld, John. *The Secret and Sublime.* New York: E. P. Dutton and Co., 1973.

Capra, F. *The Tao of Physics.* New York: Dell, 1977.

Chang, Stephen Thomas. *The Complete Book of Acupuncture.* Millbrae, CA: Celestial Arts, 1976.

Ch'ih chiao i sheng shou ts'e tr. *A Barefoot Doctor's Manual*. Philadelphia: Running Press, 1977.

Huang T., Nei Ching Su Wen. *The Yellow Emperor's Classic of Internal Medicine*. Ilza Veith, tr. Berkeley: University of California Press, 1966.

Huang, Wen-Shan. *Fundamentals of Tai Chi Ch'uan*. Hong Kong: South Sky Book Co., 1973.

Huard, Pierre, and Ming Wang. *Chinese Medicine*. New York: McGraw Hill, 1972.

Kushi, Michio. *The Book of Macrobiotics*. Japan Publications, Inc., 1977.

——. *The Macrobiotic Way of Natural Healing*. Boston: East West Publications, 1978.

Lao Tsu. *Tao Te Ching*. Gia-fu Feng and Jane English, tr. Vintage Books Edition, 1972.

Lao Tsu. *The Way of Life*. Witter Brynner, tr. New York: Capricorn Books, 1944, 15th ed. 1962.

Li Shih-Chen. *Chinese Medicinal Herbs*. San Francisco: Georgetown Press, 1973.

Lucas, Richard. *Healing Secrets of the East*. New York: Parker Publishing Co., 1980.

Maisel, Edward. *Tai Chi for Health*. New York: Delta Publications, 1963, 1972.

Mann, Felix. *Acupuncture: The Ancient Chinese Art of Healing and How It Works Scientifically*. New York: Random House, 1972.

Muramoto, Naboru. *Healing Ourselves*. Swan House Publishing Co., 1972.

Palos, Stephen. *The Chinese Art of Healing*. New York: Bantam Books, 1971.

Siu, R. G. H. *The Tao of Science: An Essay on Western Knowledge and Eastern Wisdom*. Cambridge, MA: M.I.T. Press, 1957, 1974.

Tara, William, ed., *Oriental Diagnosis from Lectures by Michio Kushi*. London: Red Moon Press, Frowde and Co., 1976.

Wilhelm, Richard, tr. *The Secret of the Golden Flower: A Chinese Book of Life*. New York: Harcourt, Brace, Jovanovich, 1970.

Zukaw, Gary. *The Dancing Wu Li Masters*. New York: Morrow and Co., 1979.

Ayurveda

Ballentine, R. M. *Diet and Nutrition.* Honesdale, PA: Himalayan Institute Press, 1978.

Bhattacharya, B. *The Science of Tridosha, an Analysis of the Three Cosmic Elements in Medicines, Food and Diseases.* New York: Gotham Book Mart, 1956.

Caraka Samhita. Jamnagar, India: Shree Gulabkunverba Ayurvedic Society, 1949.

Leslie, Charles. *Asian Medical Systems: A Comparative Study.* Berkeley: University of California Press, 1977.

Svoboda, Robert. *The Hidden Secret of Ayurveda.* India: Pune, 1980.

Thakkur, C. G. *Introduction of Ayurveda.* New York: ASI Publishers, 1974.

Philosophy Of Yoga

Ajaya, Swami. *Yoga Psychology: A Practical Guide to Meditation.* Honesdale, PA: Himalayan International Institute, 1978.

Aranya, S. Harikarananda. *Yoga Philosophy of Patanjali.* Albany: State University of New York, 1983.

Arya, Usharbudh, Ph.D. *Philosophy of Hatha Yoga.* Honesdale, PA: Himalayan International Institute, 1977.

Aurobindo, Sri. *The Synthesis of Yoga.* Pondicherry: Sri Aurobindo Ashram, 1981.

Avalon, Arthur. *The Serpent Power: The Secrets of Tantric and Shaktic Yoga.* New York: Dover Publications, 1974.

Brena, Steven, M.D. *Yoga and Medicine.* New York: Penguin Books, 1972.

Chaudhuri, Haridas. *Integral Yoga: The Concept of Harmonious and Creative Living.* Wheaton, IL: Quest Books, Theosophical Publishing House, 1925, 1974.

Chinmayananda, Swami. *Mandukya Upanishad.* Bombay: Central Mission Trust, 1953.

Coster, Geraldine. *Yoga and Western Psychology.* New York: Harper Colophon Books, 1972.

Deussen, Paul. *The System of Vedanta.* New York: Dover Books, 1912, 1973.

Funderburk, James. *Science Studies Yoga.* Honesdale, PA: Himalayan International Institute, 1977.

McDermott, Robert, ed., *The Essential Aurobindo.* New York: Schocken Books, 1973.

Naranjo, Claudio, and Robert Ornstein. *On the Psychology of Meditation.* New York: Penguin Books, 1977.

Nikhilananda, Swami (translator). *The Gospel of Sri Ramakrishna.* Sri Ramakrishna Math, India, 1969.

Prabhavananda, Swami, and Christopher Isherwood. *Shankara's Crest Jewel of Discrimination.* Los Angeles: Vedanta Press, 1978.

Rama, Swami. *Freedom from the Bondage of Karma.* Honesdale, PA: Himalayan International Institute, 1977.

_____. *Lectures on Yoga.* Honesdale, PA: Himalayan International Institute, 1979.

_____. *Living with the Himalayan Masters.* Honesdale, PA: Himalayan International Institute, 1978.

_____, Rudolph Ballentine and Swami Ajaya. *Yoga and Psychotherapy: The Evolution of Consciousness.* Honesdale, PA: Himalayan International Institute, 1976.

Vivekananda, Swami. *Jnana Yoga.* India: Advaita Ashrama, 1972.

_____. *Raja Yoga.* Ramakrishna-Vivekananda Center, 1973.

Wood, Ernest. *Yoga.* Everyday Handbooks, 1977.

Woods, J. H. *The Yoga System of Patanjali.* India: Motilal Banarsidass, 1977.

Yogananda, Paramahansa. *Autobiography of a Yogi.* Los Angeles: Self-Realization Fellowship, 1973.

Pranayama

Fletcher, Ella Adelia. *The Law of the Rhythmic Breath.* San Bernadino, CA: Bargo Press, 1980.

Kuvalayananda, Swami. *Pranayama.*

Prasad, Rama. *Nature's Finer Forces. The Science of*

Breath and the Philosophy of the Tattvas. Phoenix:
Health Research, 1894, 1969.

Rama, Swami, Rudolph Ballentine and Alan Hymes. *The Science of Breath: A Practical Guide.* Honesdale, PA: Himalayan Institute Press, 1979.

Saraswati, Swami Satyananda. *Asana Pranayama Mudra Bandha.* India: Bihar School of Yoga, 1977.

Sivananda, Swami. *The Science of Pranayama.* Divine Life Society Publications, 1971.

Van Lysebeth, Andre. *Pranayama: The Yoga of Breathing.* Vershire, VT: Mandala Books, 1979.

Hatha Yoga

Iyengar, B. K. S. *Light on Yoga.* New York: Schocken Books, 1976.

Kuvalayananda, Swami. *Popular Yoga.* Rutland, VT: Charles E. Tuttle Co., 1971.

Rieker, Hans-Ulrich. *The Yoga of Light: Hatha Yoga Pradipika.* Dawn Horse Press, 1974.

Samskriti and Judith Franks. *Hatha Yoga Manual II.* Honesdale, PA: Himalayan International Institute, 1978.

_____, and Veda. *Hatha Yoga Manual I.* Honesdale, PA: Himalayan International Institute, 1979.

Satchidananda, Swami. *Integral Yoga—Hatha.* New York: Holt Paperback, 1975.

Van Lysebeth, Andre. *Yoga Self Taught.* New York: Barnes and Noble Books, 1973.

Vishnudevananda, Swami. *The Complete Book of Illustrated Yoga.* New York: Pocket Books, 1972.

Nutrition

Aerola, Paavo. *Are You Confused.* Phoenix: Health Plus Publishers, 1971.

_____. *How to Get Well*. Phoenix: Health Plus Publishers, 1974.

Ballentine, R. M. *Diet and Nutrition*. Honesdale, PA: Himalayan Institute Press, 1974.

Birch, Herbert G., and Joan Dye Gussow. *Disadvantaged Children: Health, Nutrition, and School Failure*. New York: Grune & Stratton, 1970.

Bodwell, C., ed., *Evaluation of Proteins for Humans*. Wilport, CT: AVI Publications, 1977.

Cheraskin, E., M.D., W. M. Ringsdork, and J. L. Clark. *Diet and Disease*. New Canaan, CT: Keats Publishing, Inc., 1977.

Cleave, T. L. *The Saccharine Disease*. New Canaan, CT: Keats Publishing, Co., 1975.

Dandria, Su Stanley, et al. *Human Nutrition and Dietetics*. New York: Churchill Livingstone, 1975.

Hawkins, D., and L. Pauling, eds., *Orthomolecular Psychiatry*. San Francisco: W. H. Freeman, 1973.

Hull, Gary. *The New Vegetarian*. New York: William Morrow & Co., 1978.

Human Nutrition. (Reprints from Scientific American). San Francisco: W. H. Freeman, 1978.

Nutrition Search, Inc. *Nutrition Almanac*. New York: McGraw Hill, 1975.

Owen, George, et al. "A study of nutritional status of preschool children in the United States, 1968-1970." *Pediatrics* 53 (4, Part II): 597-646, 1974.

Pauling, L. *Vitamin C and the Common Cold*. San Francisco, CA: W. H. Freeman, 1976.

Pfeiffer, C. *Mental and Elemental Nutrients*. New Canaan, CT: Keats Publishing Co., 1975.

Randolph, T. G., L. Rosenzweig, and E. Kailin. *Food Addiction and Ecological Mental Illness*. Chicago: Human Ecology Research Foundation, 1971.

_____. *Human Ecology and Susceptibility to the Chemical Environment*. Springfield, IL: Charles C. Thomas, 1962, 1981.

Read, Merrill S. "Behavioral correlates of malnutrition". *Growth and Development of the Brain*. ed. Mary A. B. Brazier. New York: Raven Press, (In press, 1975).

Schroeder, Henry, M.D. *The Trace Elements and Man*. Old Greenwich, CT: Devin-Adair Co., 1973.

Stone, I. *The Healing Factor—Vitamin C Against Disease*. New York: Grosset and Dunlap, 1972.

Travis, J. W. *Wellness Workbook.* Mill Valley, CA:
Wellness Center, 1979.

U. S. Dept. of Agriculture. *Composition of Foods: Raw,
processed, prepared.* Agriculture Handbook No. 8.
Washington, D. C. Government Printing Office,
1963.

Watson, G. *Nutrition and your Mind.* New York: Harper
and Row, 1972.

Williams, R. J. *Biochemical Individuality.* Austin: Univ.
of Texas Press, 1969.

_____. *Nutrition Against Disease.* New York: Bantam
Books, 1973.

_____, and K. A. Dwight. *A Physician's Handbook on
Orthomolecular Medicine.* New York: Pergamon
Press, 1977.

Movement Therapy

Brena, Steven F. *Yoga and Medicine.* New York: Pelican
Books, 1973.

Brown, Barbara. *New Mind, New Body—Biofeedback:
New Directions for the Mind.* New York: Harper and
Row, 1974.

Cater, Mildred. *Helping Yourself with Foot Reflexology.*
Englewood Cliffs, NJ: Parker Publishing Co., 1969.

Cooper, K. H. *The New Aerobics.* New York: Bantam,
1975.

_____, and M. E. Cooper. *Aerobics for Women.* New
York: Bantam, 1976.

Downing, George. *The Massage Book.* New York:
Random House, 1972.

Dychtwald, Ken. *Body Mind.* New York: Jove Publishing
Co., 1977.

Felenkrais, Moshe. *Awareness through Movement.* New
York: Harper and Row, 1977.

Jacobsen, E. *Progressive Relaxation.* Chicago: University
of Chicago Press, 1929, 1974.

Johnson, Don. *The Protein Body: A Rolfer's View of
Human Flexibility.* New York: Harper Colophon
Books, 1977.

Kuvalayananda, Swami, and S. L. Vinekar. *Yoga Therapy*. India: Government of India Press, 1963, 1971.

Lowen, Alexander. *Bioenergetics*. New York: Penguin Books, 1975.

_____. *The Language of the Body*. New York: Collier Books, 1978.

_____, and Leslie Lowen. *The Way to Vibrant Health. A Manual of Bioenergetic Exercises*. New York: Harper and Row, 1977.

Luce, Gay. *Body Time*. New York: Bantam, 1973.

Montagu, Ashley. *Touching—The Human Significance of the Skin*. New York: Harper and Row, 1978.

Rolf, Ida. *Rolfing: The Integration of Human Structures*. New York: Harper and Row, 1977.

Spino, M. *Beyond Jogging*. Millbrae, CA: Celestial Arts, 1976.

Teeguarden, Iona. *Acupuncture Way of Health: Jin Shin Do*. Japan Publications, 1978.

Thie, John F. *Touch for Health*. Marina del Rey, CA: DeVorss & Co., 1979

Stress Management Therapy

Brown, Barbara. *Stress and the Art of Biofeedback*. New York: Harper and Row, 1977.

Glasser, Ronald. *The Body is the Hero*. Westminster, MD: Random House, 1976.

Green, Elmer and Alyce. *Beyond Biofeedback*. New York: Delta, 1977.

Luthe, W. *Autogenic Therapy*. New York: Grune and Stratton, 1969.

Moss, Ralph. *The Cancer Syndrome*. New York: Grove Press, 1980.

Nuernberger, Phil. *Freedom from Stress*. Honesdale, PA: Himalayan Institute, 1981.

Pelletier, Kenneth. *Mind as Healer, Mind as Slayer*. New York: Dell, 1977.

_____. *Toward a Science of Consciousness*. New York: Delta, 1978.

_____, and Charles Garfield. *Consciousness East and West*. New York: Harper Colophon, 1976.

Selye, Hans. *The Stress of Life*. New York: McGraw Hill, 1976.

Psychotherapy

Assagioli, Roberto, M.D. *Psychosynthesis*. New York: Penguin, 1976.

Fromm, Erich, D.T.S. Suzuki, and Richard Martino. *Zen Buddhism and Psychoanalysis*. New York: Harper and Row, 1970.

Jacobi, Jolande, and R.F.C. Hull. *C. G. Jung Psychological Reflection*. Bollingen Series. Princeton: Princeton Univ. Press, 1953, 1973.

James, William. *Psychology*. New York: Harper and Row, 1892, 1961.

Jung, C. G. *Psychology and the East*. Bollingen Series. Princeton: Princeton University Press, 1978.

_____. *The Collected Works of C. G. Jung*. Bollingen Series XX. Princeton: Princeton University Press, 1968.

_____, ed, *Man and His Symbols*. New York: Dell, 1964, 1978.

Krishnamurti, J. *Talks and Dialogues*. New York: Avon Books, 1976.

Laing, R. D. *The Divided Self*. New York: Penguin Books, 1969.

Laszlo, Violet, ed. *Psyche and Symbols of C. G. Jung*. New York: Doubleday Anchor Books, 1958.

Maslow, Abraham. *Motivation and Personality*. New York: Harper and Row, 1954, 1970.

_____. *The Farther Reaches of Human Nature*. New York: Penguin, 1976.

_____. *Toward a Psychology of Being*. New York: D. Van Nostrand Co., 1968.

May, Rollo, ed., *Existential Psychology*. New York: Random House, 1960, 1969.

Naranjo, Claudio, and Robert E. Ornstein. *On the*

Psychology of Meditation. New York: Esalen Books, Viking Press, 1973.

Perls, Frederick, M.D., Ph.D. *Gestalt Therapy Verbatim.* New York: Bantam Books, 1971.

Werner, Irving B. *Principles of Psychotherapy.* New York: John Wiley and Sons, 1975.

Wilson, Colin. *New Pathways in Psychology, Maslow and the Post Freudian Revolution.* New York: Mentor Books, 1972.

Whitmont, Edward. *The Symbolic Quest: Basic Concepts of Analytic Psychology.* Princeton: Princeton University Paperbacks, 1978.

Homeopathic and Medicinal Therapy

Allen, H. C., M.D. *Keynotes and Characteristics of the Materia Medica with Nosodes.* New Delhi, India: Jain Publishing Co.

Alexander, Franz, M.D. *Psychosomatic Medicine.* New York: W. W. Norton and Co., 1965.

Anderson, David, M.D., Dale Buegel, M.D., and Dennis Chernin, M.D. *Homeopathic Remedies.* Honesdale, PA: Himalayan Institute, 1978.

Bach, Edward, M.D., and F. S. Wheeler, M.S. *The Bach Flower Remedies.* New Canaan, CT: Keats Publishing, Inc., 1979.

Baker, W. P., M.D., et al. *Introduction to Homeotherapeutics.* Washington, D.C.: American Institute of Homeopathy, 1974.

Bakker. "Osteoarthritic Nosode 30c." *The British Journal of Homeopathy.* Vol. LV, No. 3, July 1966, p. 165.

Banerjee, P. N. *Chronic Disease: Its Cause and Cure.* Bengal, India: Banerjee and Co., 1971.

Blackie, Margery. *The Patient, Not the Cure. The Challenge of Homeopathy.* Santa Barbara, CA: Woodbridge Press, 1978.

Bodman. "Ulcerative Colitis and Diverticulitis." *The British Homeopathic Journal.* Vol. LXIV, No. 4, Oct. 1975, p. 201.

Boericke, William, M.D. *Pocket Manual of Homeopathic Materia Medica with Repertory*, 9th ed. Philadelphia: Boericke and Runyon, 1927.

———, and Willis Dewey, M.D. *The Twelve Tissue Remedies of Schuessler*. Philadelphia: Boericke and Tafel, 1914.

Borland, Douglas. *Children's Types*. Delhi, India: N. S. and Co.

Chapman, J. B., M.D. *Dr. Schuessler's Biochemistry, A Medical Book for the Home*. London: New Era Laboratories, LTD, 1977.

Clarke, John Henry, M.D. *A Dictionary of Practical Materia Medica*, 3 volumes. New Delhi: Jain Publishing Co., 1978.

Cooper. "The Homeopathic Treatment of Gastric Duodenal Ulceration." *The Homeopathic Recorder*, Vol. XLIV, No. 1, January 15, 1929, p. 26.

Coulter, Harris. *Divided Legacy, a History of the Schism in Medical Thought*, 3 volumes. Washington, D. C.: Wehawken Book Co., 1977.

Cox, D., and T. W. Hyne-Jones. *Before the Doctor Comes*. Rustington, Sussex, England: Health Science Press, 1974.

Dewey, W. A., M.D. *Practical Homeopathic Therapeutics*. New Delhi, India: Jain Publishing Co.

"Gastric Ulcers." *The British Homeopathic Journal*, Vol. LX, No. 2, April 1971, p. 119.

Gibson, D. M., M.D. *First Aid Homeopathy in Accidents and Ailments*. London: The British Homeopathic Association, 1975.

Goldner. "Clinical Aspects of Hypoadrenocorticism in Otolaryngology." *Journal of the American Institute of Homeopathy*, Vol. 63, No. 1, March 1970, p. 31.

Grossinger, Richard. *Planet Medicine*. Boulder, CO: Shambhala Publ., 1982.

Hahnemann, Samuel. *The Chronic Diseases: Their Peculiar Nature and Their Homeopathic Cure*. New Delhi: Jain Publishing Co., 1835, 1978.

Hering, C., M.D. *The Guiding Symptoms of our Materia Medica*. 10 vols. New Delhi, India: Jain Publishers, reprint 1974.

Kent, James Tyler, M.D. *Lectures on Homeopathic Materia Medica with New Remedies*. New Delhi, India: Jain Publishing Co., 1975.

_____. *Lectures on Homeopathic Philosophy.* New Delhi: Jain Publishers, 1st reprint 1970.

_____. *Reperatory of the Homeopathic Materia Medica with Word Index.* New Delhi: Jain Publishing Co., 6th ed., 1975.

MacNeill. "Rheumatoid Arthritis." *The British Homeopathic Journal,* Vol. LXV, No. 1, January 1977, p. 13.

Nash, E. B., M.D. *Leaders in Homeopathic Therapeutics.* Philadelphia: Boericke, and Tafel, 6th ed. 1926.

Panos, Maesimind, and Jane Heimlich. *Homeopathic Medicine at Home.* Los Angeles: J. P. Tarcher, 1981.

Pierce, Willard, M.D. *Plain Talks of Materia Medica with Comparisons.* Calcutta: Hanen and Brothers, 5th ed. 1970.

Roberts, Herbert, M.D. *Sensations as if: A Reperatory of Subjective Symptoms.* New Delhi: Jain Publishing Co., 1894, 1976.

_____. *The Principles and Art of Cure by Homeopathy.* Rustington, Sussex, England: Health Science Press, 1942.

Shepherd, Dorothy, M.D. *Homeopathy for the First Aider.* Rustington, Sussex, England: Health Science Press, 2nd ed. 1953.

_____. *Magic of the Minimum Dose.* Rustington, Sussex, England: Health Science Press, 1938, 1979.

Shippen. "Rheumatoid Arthritis; A Case Report." *Journal of the American Institute of Homeopathy,* Vol. 69, No. 1, March 1976, p. 11.

Speight, Phyllis. *A Comparison of the Chronic Miasms.* Devon, England: Health Science Press, 1977.

Stewart. "Coronary Heart Disease." *The British Homeopathic Journal,* Vol. LV, No. 3, July 1966, p. 142.

Tyler, M. L. *Homeopathic Drug Pictures.* Sussex, England: Health Science Press, 1942.

Vithoulkas, George. *Homeopathy: Medicine for the New Man.* New York: Arco Publ., 1979.

_____. *The Science of Homeopathy, a Modern Textbook,* Vol. 1. Athens: A.S.O. H. M., 1978.

Weiner, Michael. *Complete Book of Homeopathy.* New York: Bantam Books, 1981.

Whitmont, Edward. *Psyche and Substance.* Richmond, CA: North Atlantic Books, 1980.

_____. "Psychosomatics." *Journal of the American Institute of Homeopathy*, Vol. 57, No. 5-6, May-June, 1964, p. 8.

_____. "Towards a Basic Law of Psychic and Somatic Relationship," *Journal of the American Institute of Homeopathy*, Vol. 69, No. 1, March, 1976, p. 15.

Herbal Medicine

Culpepper, Nicholas. *Culpepper's English Physician and Complete Herbal.* Arranged by C. F. Leyel. Hollywood, CA: Wilshire Book Co., 1977.

Esplan, Ceres. *Herbal Teas for Health and Healing.* Northamptonshire, England: Thorson's Publishers, LTD, 1976.

Harris, Ben Charles. *The Compleat Herbal.* New York: Larchmont Books, 1972.

Kloss, Jethro. *Back to Eden.* Santa Barbara, CA: Lifeline Books, 1939, 1974.

Lust, John, M.D. *The Herb Book.* New York: Bantam Books, 1974.

Stuart, Malcolm, ed., *The Encyclopedia of Herbs and Herbalism.* New York: Grosset and Dunlap, 1979.

Anatomy and Physiology

Asimov, Isaac. *The Human Body: Its Structure and Operation.* New York: Mentor Books, 1963.

Frohse, Franz, Max Brodel, and Leon Schlossberg. *Atlas of Human Anatomy.* New York: Barnes and Noble, 1961.

Ganong, William. *Review of Medical Physiology.* Los Altos, CA: Lange Medical Publications, 1981.

Gilman, Sid, and Sarah Winans. *Manter and Gatz's. Essentials of Clinical Neuroanatomy and*

Neurophysiology. Philadelphia: F. A. Davis Co., 1982.

Gray, Henry. *Gray's Anatomy*. Philadelphia: Running Press, 1901, 1973.

Halvey, David, M.D., ed., *The Merck Manual of Diagnosis and Therapy*. Rahway, NJ: Merck and Co., 1972.

Jacob, Stanley, M.D., and Clarice Francone. *Structure and Function in Man*. Philadelphia: Saunder's Co., 1978.

Kempe, Henry, Henry Silver, and Donough O'Brien, eds. *Current Pediatric Diagnosis and Treatment*. Los Altos, CA: Lange Medical Publications, 1982.

Murray, I. MacKay. *Human Anatomy Made Simple*. New York: Doubleday and Co., 1969.

Vander, Arthur, James Sherman, and Dorothy Luciano. *Human Physiology: the Mechanisms of Body Function*. New York: McGraw Books Co., 1975.

Wintrobe, Maxwell, M.D., et al. *Harrison's Principles of Internal Medicine*. New York: McGraw Hill, 1980.

Woodburne, Russell. *Essentials of Human Anatomy*. New York: Oxford University Press, 1978.

About the Authors

Dennis K. Chernin, M.D., practices holistic medicine in Ann Arbor, Michigan. A graduate of the University of Michigan Medical School, he was a psychiatric resident at the University of Wisconsin. He is on the faculty at the Himalayan Institute of Yoga Science and Philosophy and has taught classes in homeopathy and meditation at the University of Michigan (extension), and he is currently finishing a Masters of Public Health there. Dr. Chernin is co-author of the book *Homeopathic Remedies*.

Gregory Manteuffel, M.D., a graduate of Wayne State Medical School, has studied and taught homeopathy for six years. A holistic family practitioner, he is currently medical director at the Hering Family Health Clinic in Berkeley, California.

Index